A PAST LIFE:
as told by Brave Hawk

DonD Sylvain

A Past Life: as told by Brave Hawk by DonD Sylvain

This book is written to provide information and motivation to readers. Its purpose isn't to render any type of psychological, legal, or professional advice of any kind. The content is the sole opinion and expression of the author, and not necessarily that of the publisher.

Copyright © 2020 by DonD Sylvain

All rights reserved. No part of this book may be reproduced, transmitted, or distributed in any form by any means, including, but not limited to, recording, photocopying, or taking screenshots of parts of the book, without prior written permission from the author or the publisher. Brief quotations for noncommercial purposes, such as book reviews, permitted by Fair Use of the U.S. Copyright Law, are allowed without written permissions, as long as such quotations do not cause damage to the book's commercial value. For permissions, write to the publisher, whose address is stated below.

ISBN: 978-1-952617-56-0 (Paperback)
ISBN: 978-1-64934-132-7 (Hardback)
Printed in the United States of America

Rustik Haws LLC
100 S. Ashley Drive, Suite 600
Tampa, FL 33602
https://www.rustikhaws.com/

We lived by a river that had a large floodplain, it had very rich soil. The farm was on a rise of ground overlooking the river and flood plain. The farm was located south west of what is now Lake Michigan. My grandparents and my father and mother established the farm. My grandparents are now deceased. My father Mark and my mother Mary and Aunt Sue now ran the farm. Chum my older brother and I were always busy at chores, trapping, fishing and hunting.

Our farm was located a mile and a half or so from the village. We hired help from the village at times. We also had living quarters for our workers who help run the farm. We had cows, horses and chickens. We didn't raise hogs. The villagers raised hogs and if we wanted any pork we would barter for it. We also had a pair of wonderful black mules. They were very strong and did a lot of the heavy work hauling a wagon and doing the plowing etc. We had a large wagon also two wheel carts with very large wheels. The wagon and carts were used to haul our goods for trade into the city our house was located next to a spring that ran year around. Our water was always clear and easily accessible. Our house had plank flooring. The houses in the village were all dirt floors at this time. I didn't realize at the time, we were quite well-to-do. Our house was much larger than any others, it was surprising for me to go into the houses in the village and find dirt floors. I did this on occasion to deliver papers or some other things to the family. I didn't know why but there didn't seem to be many small children or babies in the village. All the girls were married or seem to be attached to someone. This didn't seem to bother Chum or I. We had so many other interests to keep us busy when our chores were done such as fishing hunting trapping and exploring.

When younger, Chum and I weren't very keen on learning. Mom and dad insisted and would tutor us with Susan's help. It wasn't long we started to read some of the books that my father had in his library then Chum and I were glad we had been made to study. Mother and father were well educated, were the only ones

A Past Life: as told by Brave Hawk

who could read and write in this area. This was also a good source of income, villagers from all over came to them for reading of letters and legal papers etc. Mother and Aunt Sue were herbalist and many came to them for healing herbs which was another source of income.

Aunt Sue was my father's younger sister she wasn't a lot older than I was. Aunt Sue took me under her wing and kept track of me and my shenanigans. I was an only child, I thought a boy named Chum was my older brother but he wasn't a brother by blood, he was adopted. We got along very well and did everything together. I was called Bird because of all my tumbling and running antics. Mother said I was like a bird flitting and landing here and there. I would light and perch on the rail fence that went around mother's herb garden. Then I would run along the rails and this is when mother said I was acting like a little bird. This is when everybody started calling me bird. I don't recall my real name.

I loved the mules and I was around them all the time. I was under their feet a lot, would also run and tumble and light on their backs. Chum and my father didn't know how the mules put up with me. My father watched, could see that the mules were very careful not to step on me. Father concluded that the mules really like me as I did them.

Every evening after chores Chum and I had to study, reading writing arithmetic etc. Then we had sponge baths before bed, mother insisted. Mom dad aunt Sue, then Chum and I would take clean water in a large basin for our sponge bath. This consisted of washing the whole body. Mom would have different herbs that smelt real good, so we went to bed smelling fresh. In the mornings we washed our hands and face. Then had breakfast, eggs and porridge and meat. Milk was our main drink at breakfast and at evening meals.

We were now ready for our chores. When younger my chores consisted of gathering the eggs cleaning the hen house. I kind of enjoyed this. My Aunt Sue would assist me, it was a good experience. Sue would show me how to get the eggs from under a sitting hen. She would wave one hand in front of the hen then slide the other hand under the hen and retrieve the eggs. Chum and I also had to watch for fox, raccoons and skunks etc. We made traps and caught quite a few. The hides were worth a good sum so they were sent to the city. As I grew older, my chores increased to working with Chum and others in the sheds and barn. This is when I was around the animals cows, horses and the mules. This was a lot of enjoyment for me also. Learning how to handle animals without getting hurt and without hurting them.

Chum had a horse of his own. Mom at first wanted to get me a pony, but dad had different ideas. He ended up buying me a filly. We became very attached. Chum and I were together all the time. He was my big brother, he would laugh at my tumbling and cartwheels. He and dad really enjoyed how the mules put up with my antics.

Dad Hired a strange man who came looking for work. We had a large plot of land that dad wanted to plow so the mules were harnessed and brought out to the plot. The mules just would not work for this man. I was keeping an eye on the mules, I could tell the mules didn't like this man at all. Next thing that happened, the man went into the woods and got a large stick, he was going to beat the mules. This is when I ran and put a stop to it. I then ran and got on one of the mules back. They then behaved only because I was there. At noon I went looking for my father, then told him how the man was acting around the mules. He was going to beat the mules and I put a stop to it. Then I got on the mules back and stayed till lunchtime. Dad got rid of the man and paid for a day's wages. Then he said any man that treats an animal in that fashion isn't much of a man.

As I grew older Chum taught me about the Flint lock Rifle. Dad found one for me from the blacksmith and gunsmith in the village.

A Past Life: as told by Brave Hawk

I knew the blacksmith and gunsmith by the name of Chuck. The rifle dad chose for me was one of Chuck's designs. It was shorter and lighter and a little easier to handle. I travelled with Chum with a rifle before. So knew what was going on with the hunting and fishing. This was a new experience for me, first time I was actually shooting at an animal. Had done a lot of practicing before I was allowed to hunt. Safety was always the first thing I was taught. I became a real good shot, Chum was also a good shot. We competed he would out shoot me then I would out shoot him.

When we had planned on hunting, next day, we didn't shirk our chores. But worked like heck to get our chores done. Then we were off on our next excursion. At the time hunting and fishing and trapping were year-round. When we managed to bring back fish and game mom and Aunt Sue were happy to cook them for everyone's meal. The hides from trapping were cleaned and ship to the city. We used salt to preserve them.

I don't recall any church but we always said prayers at meals and in the evenings. At one time a preacher came to the village and everyone was enthused to be able to hear some preaching, prayers and hymns to sing to. Mom, Dad, Aunt Sue, Chum and I went to the village to hear this preacher. It was an outdoor arrangement, the villagers had set up rough benches and others just sat on the ground. Mom and Sue had made lunches for all. The preacher showed up with his Bible he didn't say any prayers, but started in with fire and brimstone type of hollering and if everybody didn't listen to them they were going to hell. My father then stood up and motioned to mom, Sue Chum and myself it was time to go. I could tell dad was really upset. As we left the preacher followed used words that were quite offensive to dad. Dad turned and faced the preacher and proceeded to walk him backwards. When he saw the look on dad's face the preacher backed off. When dad and our family left many of the villagers did also. Mom and dad are well respected in the village and all around. They knew dad was very upset with this preacher.

Chuck the gunsmith and his two-men hadn't come to the meeting. The villagers proceeded to tell him what had happened. They told how upset dad was and how the preacher carried on. Even after dad left he was saying that dad and everybody else would to go to hell because they weren't listening. He also was telling everyone our family was sure to experience the wrath of God. When he had finished everyone left.

Chuck and his two men went looking for the preacher. It wasn't long before they found him. They then just gathered them up, took him to a tree, then put a rope around his neck through it over a limb and hauled it uptight. The preacher was so scared he even wet himself. He was then told if they let them go and that he was found anywhere in the vicinity they would hang him. He left in one hurry, and was never seen again.

Chum and I were spending a lot of time at the blacksmith shop. Chuck had a couple of men working for him, he did all the supervising, the finer work he took care of himself. I was interested in the shop especially the rifles and their works. Chuck was about my mother's age. His mother and father were both dead. His father left him the blacksmith shop and all the tools. Chuck had left to go back east for a while. He would tell us about some of his exploits. He was always welcome at our house and was very good friends with mom and dad. I asked about his mother and he said he didn't remember her. She had crossed over when he was very young. When he returned from his gallivanting he was ready to settle down, and resumed working with his father in the shop. He told us that his father passed away shortly after he had returned home.

Chuck would come to dinner once a week or sometimes more. Chum and I really enjoyed his talk with father and mother and we would get him to tell about his shenanigans when he was back east. He was in with a rough bunch and learned how to handle himself in a fight. It wasn't long before no one challenged him.. He was that good.

A Past Life: As Told By Brave Hawk

On Sundays the villagers would have contest of all kinds. Running, shooting, wrestling etc, no one could beat me at running. I was always way out front in every race. They decided to put in obstacles to slow me down, but it just slowed the others down. I would make tumbling jumps over most and hand vault over the real tall ones. Chum and I would also enter their shooting contest, we were both excellent shots. One time Chum would out shoot me, the next time I would out shoot him. Very seldom we would not fail to win the prize. The prizes were usually cooked food goods of some kind. Apples potatoes and any other vegetables like beets, carrots, squash, pumpkins etc.. Cakes and pies were the favorites. Mom and dad furnished a lot of the prizes. There was a lot of drinking, but overall everyone had a good time.

Bow shooting was another contest I didn't participate in. I would stand at the targets and confirm where the arrow struck. While doing this I could see arrows coming, and I told others that you could knock an arrow out of the air because I could see them coming. Best if you stand at the side of the arrows path. They just laughed at me. So I stood next to the target and proceeded to knock an arrow out of the air before it hit the target. The Bowman was very angry. I apologized, and told him that the Guys laughed at me so I was bound to prove it could be done. He was also amazed that I was able to do it. I promised to replace his arrow with more than just one. This satisfied him.

The only time there was trouble was when strangers showed up. Most just enjoyed the challenges and fun. Chuck and a few others kept things in hand. A bully showed up, he had challenged and beat up some of the contestants. He used this stick club in his fighting. Chuck had been keeping an eye on him, this is when Chuck got Chum and I together told us we needed to know how to protect ourselves in a fight. He said this bully had been watching me and knew he would look for an opportunity to corner and challenge me. Like Chuck said he couldn't be by my side all the time when the bully was around. Chuck said it might not happen, but being prepared was assurance of not getting beaten to a pulp. Chuck worked with Chum and I out back in his blacksmith shop, he showed us a lot of is fighting strategies. One main thing was not to hit so much but to poke real hard instead. He also said take your jacket or shirt and wrap it around your arm to ward off the main part of the blow. Always anticipate the blow that was coming ward it off and make your move at the same time. Don't hesitate, if possible always attack first. This gives a much greater advantage when you get in the first blow. After a couple weeks we were pretty darn good. Chum and I had fun practicing together. We were enjoying life and spent all our time together.

It wasn't half a dozen Sundays that went by when I got challenge I had started carrying a club of my own design in my waistband. I left the gathering to get some cold water from the spring. This is when this bully and his followers cornered me. I had turned to go back to the village games and six of these Guys were standing there. This bully had a mean smirk on his face. I then wrapped my arm with my shirt before I was quite ready, he came at me. I warded his blows off with my arm, he saw his blow were being caught by my arm and decided to go for my legs. Then I was able to get a good jab in his left side as he stooped to hit my legs. I was still able to ward off that blow with my arm. My Jab had taken some of the wind out of him. He then struck again, checked it with my arm. I then made a hell of a jab to his upper gut. This stopped him dead in his tracks. Then I jabbed him in the throat. When he grabbed his throat, I stepped in and gave a hard wallop to the side of the head, which put him down. He dropped his club so I went over and picked it up. The fight had lasted about five minutes. The group that had been watching parted as I approach them. Chum heard the running was about to start, this is when someone told him the bully had challenged me and Chum took off on the run to help me, if I had needed help. I Could See Chum Coming on the Run, I met him and said I was OK but the bully wasn't. He slapped me on the back and congratulated me. The other men went to where the games were being held and told a story about the fight that was

A Past Life: as told by Brave Hawk

quite exaggerated. All I could think of it was great to have a big brother. Everyone had heard about the fight by this time and came to check me out. They thought I would have some very bad bruises to my head and face. They then found out the bully had left. He couldn't talk and was bent over holding his gut. I took the bully's club dropped it off at the blacksmith shop. I knew Chuck would know what it meant.

We went back to the village to check everything out and enjoy the rest of the afternoon. Running races were coming up and I didn't want to miss it. Chum had already won the wrestling match and would also run but he was just an average runner. I ran the races and won all events quite easily. Neither of us would do any drinking of the liquor or hard drinks. We didn't like what it did to the men that did drink also didn't like the taste. A lot of them drank to excess and by evening a good many of them had passed out. This didn't appeal to Chum or myself. Chuck would have a drink or two but never would drink to excess.

I Asked Chum where mom and dad were? Chum said they had already gone home. So we decided to go home also. I walked into the house and asked mom to look at my arm because I was having hard time moving my hand. My arm was swelled up from warding off the bully's blow. Mom said it wasn't broken just badly bruised. Thanks to Chuck's advice it was wasn't broken. My father came to see what was happening and Mom was using spring water as a compress. Dad took a look, turned and went to get his rifle down, he said to Mom he would back in a while. He thought the bully would be in the village bragging, he was going to go and shoot him. Chum chimed in with mom not to go, Chum then told dad that the bully had left in very bad shape because I beat him very badly. I had never seen my father get upset like that before, I realize then how much our father mother cared for us. I decided to carry a, stick my left shoulder. Both Dad and Chum were laughing at me and said, well Bird you are now ready for anything. Well my answer was by gosh I am ready. I knew there was no swearing aloud. We never heard dad swear and he didn't condone it. So we never fell in the habit of doing it.

Fall was just starting and it wouldn't be long before we had to start cutting the wheat. This is done with a scythe. I would do my best to outdo Chum at this, but he was always way ahead of me. He got a big kick out of beating me. He would say, Bird this is the only thing I can outdo you at. That wasn't really true but he did not want to hurt my feelings. It didn't really bother me, we were too close to ever have hard feelings between us.

One morning dad said, well boys time to get ready, the wheat is dry and it's time to harvest it. We also had other gatherings to do in the fields that had been planted with different crops. Chum and I harnessed the mules and started out. Even though my arm was real sore, I wasn't about to neglect my chores. I really enjoyed working with Chum and dad. Dad would join us shortly. He also liked getting out into the fields, we had other help who stayed in the other small houses. They were working in the barn threshing the wheat we brought in. Dad joined us the field shortly. We had been working only about an hour or so, we saw dad go over and lean on the wagon wheel. Chum and I thought he was taking a break, he then slumped down to the ground. This is when we knew something was wrong, we raced over to dad. He was laying very still, Chum said I will stay go get mom. Mom came on the run with me. She knelt down beside dad and found he had no heartbeat. He had crossed over .This was very hard on all of us. We then went got help and brought dad into the house. At times mom and Sue had helped others that had crossed over in preparing them for burial. But our cook and the other woman that work for us took over and prepared dad for burial. Someone had went to the village and informed everybody at the village what had happened. Chuck showed up shortly and he pretty much supervised what needed to be done. Dad was well-liked by most everyone so a lot of people showed up. Wake lasted three days. Was very hard on mom and Sue. Chum and I were devastated also. Took a lot out of the household and our help.

Dad was buried on a rise of ground some distance in the back of the house. Chum and I knew someone else was buried there, we didn't know who. This is when Chum and I learned, from Aunt Sue who had been buried there. Both my mom and fathers parents were buried there. Also other babies and were born that didn't survive, were also buried there. This is also when Chum and I learned that Sue was dad's younger sister. Sue had had a few suitors but none appealed to her. She had one that she was interested in. He was killed in some type of accident. So she turned down all other suitors. She said she'd rather be alone than have to go through another tragedy. Sue was great with Mom whom I hadn't seen cry, but knew she had in privacy. Mom and dad had been very close. I also learned that I had other siblings that had died and were also buried there. Mom or dad had never related any of this to me or Chum. We had never been curious enough to ask. Sue was the one who filled us in. She said it was too hard for mom and dad to talk about it. This is why they cared so much for Chum and I, but were unwilling to spoil us. Mom and dad had made sure we could read and write. Chum and I did enjoy reading a lot of dad's books. Mom and dad also gave us a lot of freedom to hunt fish and trap. Trapping was quite profitable, the hides went to the city for sale.

Chum and I didn't have the experience to supervise the farm. Mom was very good at it, but it took her away from the things she enjoyed, her herbal garden and healing. This is when Chuck stepped in and took over, mom also asked Chuck if he would teach Chum and me the blacksmith trade. Chuck was more than willing. We then spent a lot of time at the blacksmith shop. Chum worked with the heavy work and I liked the rifle and knife making and making horseshoes to fit different horses when they came through the area.

The farm was going quite well, two men and their wives living in the cabin that had been built for this purpose.

Chum and I started working at the blacksmith shop. Chuck did not let his men go because he knew we weren't permanent. I worked on rifles and also with Chum in the shop with the other men to learn the trade. The men working in the shop were very good to Chum and me. They could have been mean and not shown us anything. Both were jolly and would pull pranks on us and laugh and give us a good nature slap on the back when we realized there were pulling our leg. They then showed us the proper way to do things. I did a lot of turning on my rifle, slim d it down to be lighter. Shooting it with heavy charges to make sure the barrel didn't rupture. I then made loads with paper so you could have the same amount of powder in each charge. The ball is also wrapped in the end of the paper. After a lot of experimenting it worked out quite well. Chuck was impressed with my work, I had also been repairing other rifles. This was the only blacksmith shop for many miles in any direction so we always had quite a bit to do.

I started to make knives, made quite a few before getting the hang of forging them properly. This is when I decided to make a larger knife to carry on my left shoulder, instead of the heavy stick I was carrying. With a lot of work and suggestions from the men in the shop, I forged out a knife that wasn't real heavy but would stand up to quite a lot of abuse, such as chopping branches and splitting kindling wood to make a fire. I also made a belt knife for gutting and skinning to replace the one I usually carried. Then I made a small knife with about 3 1/2 inch blade for cutting fingernails, toenails also if and when I needed to shave, this knife blade folded into the handle.

Chum and I still enjoyed the village games but we enjoyed our hunting and fishing much more. So when the villagers complained about a large bear they weren't able to find and kill, we decided to hunt it. This bear had killed a couple of pigs and carried off a calf. Chum and I started to track him down he was using two runways going into a swamp, about a mile and a half from the village. No one was about to go into the swamp to get the bear. So we made up plans and set up on both runways. We made a small lean-to out of pine boughs and set them up overlooking the runways. We then made our plans.

The bear was doing all his foraging at night, so just at dusk, Chum took one runway and I took the other. We had made pine lean'tos to sit in. I was really enjoying the night sounds, mice and other small animals were scurrying around. Heard an owl hoot, then heard him grab something in the leaves. I had my rifle on my lap ready to go. I dozed off, then suddenly I was wide awake. Was a beautiful evening the moon was shining so it wasn't hard to see. I knew something had awakened me, so I just sat and waited for more sound, and cocked my rifle. The next thing that happened, was the bear was right there he had heard the click of my rifle. He then made a swipe through the pine boughs with his paw, caught me across my left shoulder and chest. I was fortunate to have my rifle in the cocked position. I fired and caught the bear in the throat and he fell almost on top of me. My ball had hit him in the neck and pretty much paralyzed him. His threshing and roaring could be heard from a long ways away. Chum came on the run, he thought the bear had me down and was mauling me. I was reloading my rifle when Chum came up, took a look and finished the bear off by shooting him in the head. Chum then asked me what had happened. I told him I had dozed off and the bear had awakened me, he had come up on the side of the lean to and swiped through the pine boughs and caught me on the arm and chest. This is when Chum could see my torn shirt and could see the blood. His next comment was were going home right now. I said what about the bear. His comment was to hell with the bear, we got to get you fixed up. On the way on the trail, Chum commented some of the villagers may have heard the commotion the bear was making. Will talk back and forth just in case someone is coming so they will know it's us not the bear. Sure enough two men were coming up with rifles ready. They heard us and when we met we let them know the bear was down. He told them I was injured and was on the way home get patched up. They then said don't worry about the bear we will skin and butcher it for you. I was still bleeding quite a lot and Chum wanted to carry me, I would have none of it, I just kept plugging along. Took a shortcut to the farm. Someone from the village had gone" and woke Mom and Aunt Sue up. They told mom and Sue they had heard the bear making a lot of noise and commotion. They were worried the bear had gotten Chum or me. They said they heard the bear making a lot of roaring, then heard a shot and the bear quit roaring. They told Mom two men went to look and were afraid the bear had gotten one of us. Shortly after that Chum and I showed up. Mom took a look as I walked in. She had me sit down, then she removed by torn shirt. She proceeded to clean the wounds and apply her healing magic. Then she had me move my arm in all directions. She then told me no muscles were torn. She said, you will have scars but no muscle damage. Mom said I was really fortunate to escape without a lot more damage. I would end up with some large scars where the skin had been torn with the bear's claws.

The villagers were very grateful the bear was gone. They skinned and butchered it and brought it to the house. I asked Chum, mom and Sue if it was okay to give the bear to the villagers. Everyone thought it was a good idea.

When the men had skinned and butchered the bear they had found two bullet holes. They said they had only heard one shot. Then I told them when the bear and swiped through the lean-to my rifle was ready and I had poked into his neck and fired. That must have muffled the first shot.

Chuck was back East getting blacksmith supplies. He would've wanted to be in our escapade. When he returned and heard our story, his comment was always give yourself plenty of vision. Don't block your side view. He then said you've already learned that the hard way. He did agree that we had set up properly, except for not allowing for better side view.

Chuck now returned to the farm supervising. He knew he could trust the two men working for him at the blacksmith shop.

A Past Life: as told by Brave Hawk

Chum and I had also been working at the blacksmith shop. Chuck knew Chum and I had never been back East with the produce we had to sell and trade. He then asked mom if it would be all right for Bird and Chum to make the next trip into the city. He would keep an eye on us and direct us wherever we needed to go. Chuck was pretty city wise, he knew his way around the city. He had been in the lot a rough places and knew how to handle himself. He was well respected by the traders and other businessmen that he had things to do with, also the banks.

The next trip we loaded the wagon and one of the large wheel carts. We would trade for salt and other commodities we needed. The traveling would be 5 to 8 days going in the same coming back. This would depend on the conditions of the road in our travel. If no problems were encountered we travelled from light to dark, eating mornings and evenings.

Mom knew Chum and I had never been around any woman so mom told us to stay clear. She told us they weren't very clean about themselves and would make you very sick, maybe not right off but not to far in the future. Chuck also took us inside and told us stay clear of these woman as they were not very clean about themselves.

At this time it was slow going the roads weren't much more than trails. When we got to the city Chum and I were spellbound not being in the city before. In the more affluent part of the city, the houses were very large some of them were quite close together. In the rougher part of town the houses were very close together. We were approached by quite a few different woman selling their wares. Chuck ran them off telling them not to bother us or suffer the consequences.

Chuck did all the trading. Hard commodities were well received and Chuck knew how to watch for someone trying to cheat. He knew all the tricks, he said he had used some of them himself and laughed. Chuck also knew a good place to eat and was always welcome. They knew Chuck quite well from his traveling and trading. During his trading he showed us where the blacksmith shop was. Then he introduced us to the workers there. They then had a very large shop and it was quite interesting for us to wander around. Chum and I got different ideas just looking at all their equipment. They were using the waterwheel, actually two of them. This ran the whole mill.

When we ended up getting back to the hotel Chuck said he was going to take a bath at one of the bath houses. So we thought this would be a good idea to. Chum and I had never seen a tub before. Everyone seemed to know we were from the farm. Chuck went to the proprietor and made some kind of an agreement and then he disappeared. Then we made an agreement with the proprietor. Gave him our coin he showed us where to hang our clothes. We kept On our underclothes, not being used to being naked around other men. The next thing that happened was a man got out of the tub and we were told to get in. No way was Chum and I going to get into a dirty tub. The proprietor seen how upset we were. We demanded our coin back. We started to redress and found our knife's missing. They didn't take my large knife it was too hard to conceal. We were really angry and the proprietor gave us our coin back. He wasn't going to at first but we made such a stink that he decided not to argue. I don't believe he knew that we were with Chuck.

When Chuck came he was all spruced up. We told him that we had seen and weren't about the bathe in someone else's water, how he could we wanted to know. Chuck laughed to split a gut. He then told us he had made a deal with proprietor and tub was clean and fresh hot water was in the tub. Another lesson learned by Chum and myself.

This was in the rougher part of the city where all trading and shipping went on. I was carrying a knife on my left shoulder instead of the stick I had carried before. Chuck knew a lot of the people in the area. Because I was small boned compared to a lot of the men

A Past Life: as told by Brave Hawk

in the area, Chuck started a rumor that I was a hell of a fighter and no one was to mess with me. He also said I had the scars to prove it. Just ask the proprietor at the bathhouse. Of course the scars were from my encounter with the bear. Chum and I were together all the time. The two of us were intimidating enough so no one bothered us. Most wouldn't even approach Chum or I.

Chum and I didn't drink, so we shunned the liquor houses. After one of our evening meals, Chuck took us to a theater where the actors put on different skits. Chum and I were flabbergasted, never seeing anything like it before. We went every chance we got. I couldn't wait to get back home to tell mom and my aunt Sue about all the things we were seeing. The only thing we disliked terribly was the stink of the city. Some places were like open sewers. Chum and I enjoyed the trip to the city especially the show skits that were acted out. We very much enjoyed the blacksmith shop also, we had planned on returning to see more of it. We also seen a sawmill, decided that we should have one. So we made plans to build, somewhere not too far from the farm. Chuck still had business to finish in the city. He hired two guards because he heard there is robbing going on the trail. Some people had been killed in their goods stolen. These two men are well trusted by Chuck. They were very rough characters but very pleasant to be around. This was one of their jobs that they did. They had escorted others and had no problems.

We packed up and headed back to the farm, guides keeping a close watch. At night they took turns guarding our goods and us. We got back to the farm without any problems, the men were amazed at our farm. They stayed with us a couple days but were anxious to get back to the city. This is where their work was. Chum and I couldn't imagine living in the city.

The air and the smell of the farm and the barn smelled like perfume to us after getting the smell of the city. Now back from the trip to the city. Chum and I had watched a sawmill at work. It was run by a water wheel. We were very excited about building our own. The farm had a wonderful stream that ran year around. We would have to build a flume to guide the water to the waterwheel. Chuck said we could make some of the things we needed in the blacksmith shop. We would dicker for anything else. We needed when we went to the city. We had hand saws and axes and adz to make the beams. The hired hands would take care the farm work and do our chores. Also. Chum and I would start the building of the flume to the place where we would put the mill. The saw was a 5 foot blade that went up and down when hooked to an eccentric wheel and arm. Chuck said we could make the wheel, but he would pick up a saw blade. The next trip into the city. The road was getting better, the mud holes are filled in by each traveller. It took us less time that we had figured on. The flume was done. We then went to work on the waterwheel. This was quite large 8 foot with 2 foot buckets on it. This also went quite well. Using metal strapping were needed for strength and support. We used a 6 inch log for the actual shaft we had a lot of fun getting it straight. We used makeshift lathe to turn it straight at first we use leather lined wood for bearings, tallow for lubricant. The first time we open the flume it work fine. We hired help to make the building also had help in setting up our saw blade. When the farm's hands, chores were caught up. They came up and helped us also. With their help, things went much faster. We made our own can't hooks and peeves. Chuck did a lot of the supervising. He had liked the idea. So he got right into it. We would have boards and planks for sale before long, we also plan on making shingles. The mill was up and running before the year was out made quite a few improvements as we went along. The carriage was a challenge to get it working right. We use a rope on a drum to draw the log into the blade. A lot more work keeping things running. Then we had anticipated. Chuck knew once it was built we would lose interest. He had already planned on hiring men to run the mill and shingle makers.

The village had grown a lot. There were always some men looking for work. Chuck was a good judge of men and had hired some that were very reliable. Wasn't long were selling boards and planks most of the houses that had dirt floors. Now water playing floors. So business was brisk. Chuck took things in trade. He knew he could sell or trade in the city. He would trade for wheel castings for the carriage also a main shaft of metal for the waterwheel. Chum and I had enjoyed the challenge of getting everything to work properly.

Chum and I getting back home were enjoying the farm and the woods. Chum and I got back into a routine of hunting and fishing and trapping but still didn't shirk our farm chores. We also spent a lot of time at the blacksmith shop and getting very good at the jobs, Chuck assigned us our jobs .I was doing a lot of the rifle work. Chum did some, but preferred working in the shop with the other two men.

Chuck was now back in the farm and at every evening meal. One night he got me and Chum off to the side and then I heard him clear his throat. We had never seen him act this way before. He was always very decisive and always knew the right thing to do. Finally he blurted out he would like to ask mom to marry him. He wanted to know if we had any objections. Both Chum and I were very happy about this, we could see mom really liked Chuck. He said he had not asked as yet he wanted our okay first. This made Chum and I feel good that he would ask us first. We always had looked up to him and this made us appreciate him more. Chuck asked mom and she accepted his proposal. Sue then came and asked us what we thought. This is when we told her Chuck had already approached us and we were very happy about this marriage. Aunt Sue was visibly relieved she said she could really see them together for a long time but was afraid we would be unhappy about the union. She gave us each a hug and surprised the heck out of Chum and me. She had never shown this kind of affection before. We thought it was great, this is when I got the shock of my life, Chum said he would marry my aunt in a heartbeat. I then realize that since Chum had no direct relation to her this marriage could happen.

Sue was somewhat older than Chum still not much difference. She was probably two years older. Knowing Chums feelings, I then started to make plans to get them together. So I employed Chuck's help. He knew they liked each other very much. I had never paid any attention before, now I started watching. My aunt went out of her way to wait on Chum at meals and other little things. I realize Sue wasn't really that much older than Chum. I found out Chum was at this time 18my aunt was 20 I got after Chum sit down and have a talk with aunt Sue. He was too shy would not do it, I finally got enough nerve up to approach my aunt when we were gathering the eggs. I still helped Sue once in a while, I enjoyed the chickens and the hens. The first thing I asked if she knew how much Chum liked her. I got no reply. I then said Chum had told me he would marry you in a heartbeat. Sue looked at me and I thought she was going to cry. I started to apologize, the last thing I wanted to do was hurt her feelings. She said oh no she was glad I had told her. She was crying because she was so happy. She also said she was older and had thought Chum would look at this is a detriment. I then asked her if it would be all right to inform Chum. She agreed without hesitation the next chance I got, I told Chum he must talk to Sue, she felt the same way about him. All Chum could say was you talked to her about me? I said you know how much you like her, well she feels the same way about you. Talk to her, he finally got up his nerve and asked Sue to marry him. Sue and Chum also decided to marry, at the same time as Chuck and mom.

Marriages were performed at the farmhouse. We didn't actually go to any church meeting. There was not any church in the village. Just close friends were invited, still a good gathering. Everyone had a good time, one of the men in the village played banjo, another played the violin. So there was dancing, and a lot of socializing everyone was dressed in their Sunday best. Tobacco smoke wasn't too heavy so it's quite good. Most of the men smoked pipes so it wasn't so much of a problem. Mom or Sue wouldn't allow any chewing of tobacco in the house. So some of the men went outside to take their chew. They knew how strict mom and Sue were against

A Past Life: as told by Brave Hawk

tobacco in the house. So they went out near the barn to do their chewing.

Sleeping in the loft alone now seem weird, Chum and I had shared the loft for years. Quite a change in the household with Chuck moving in with mom and Sue moving in with Chum. I felt lost for a while. I was 16 when Chuck and Chum married. I began to daydream about going West to trade with the Indians. The farm, sawmill and blacksmith shop were doing quite well, but I felt I would like to do something that was my idea. I had not brought up the subject yet, so I told them I was daydreaming about going West setting up a trading post with the Indians. When I brought the subject of no one had any comment at first. I proceeded to tell them how we would go about this adventure. Mom chuckled and said, I knew you would want to make some kind of adventure. The farm and the village has gotten too tame for you. Chuck and Chum also thought it a great idea. Then we began to plan how and what to take on our first outing. We decided to take two wheel cart with very large wheels. From past experience we found they were much easier to haul over rough terrain" and would still carry a good load. We decided to take two canoes also, our canoes were made of cedar ash and hides that were well oiled with tallow. The tallow was also used to grease the wheels of our carts. So, I made up plans and tried to lay out the things that we needed to set up outposts. The main thing was to get a building up. We would need axes saws drills etc., which we made ourselves. I knew I would need Chuck and Chum's input if it was going to happen. Also being married might be a problem, but after some debate mom and Sue agreed it would be a good adventure and also profitable in the future. All three of us would try to keep things as light as possible, I showed them my plan and they also came up with things we would need to get started. We knew crossing any rivers would be a hazard, so the two canoes would be a bonus. The carts were built with box form so they would float without a heavy load in them. A lot of rope just for pulling and also tie downs. We tried the carts in the River and found they would float quite easily. The canoes would carry a lot of our supplies across the rivers we may have to cross.

We may have to make a few trips across any large river. We would take three draft horses and switch off each day with the hauling. Mom and thought we would take the mules. We talked it over decided to take three work horses and our mounts the mules were so used to the farm we didn't want to cause them a lot of stress, we all loved those mules. We would also take a couple of extra mounts.

With all our planning we still decided to wait till the next year to start out after the spring rains had gone by. We didn't want to contend with a spring flooding. We felt it would take 3 to 4 weeks of traveling to find a place to set up our trading post.

When the spring rains and flooding let up, we decided to try our luck at traveling. I was really excited about the trip I knew we were South West of a very large lake and we would have to cross a larger river. Not sure how many more we would have to cross. We thought we could make up from 20 to 40 miles a day if everything went well. Chuck and Chum said that if things go wrong, we would just turn around and go back home. They also may ed me agree to this. We travelled almost 3 1/2 weeks, without any serious problem. Our planning had worked out well, our tools or merchandise came out all just fine. We found a spot that was very promising near a good stream with a lot of timber for building. It wasn't long before we started putting up a large building with horses dragging the logs, and with our tools continually kept sharp things went smoothly. Making wooden shingles for the roof was tedious work. We split logs about 3 feet long into strips 10 to 12 inches wide. We started at the bottom and overlap each one to fit, we had brought some homemade nails for this purpose. The logs were drilled and pegged together wherever needed. For Windows we would use hides for lighting. Glass was very expensive and too hard to manage to keep from getting broken on our travels. Mom and dad had the only glass windows back in our village. We used hides for doors temporarily until we could have the time to saw boards out of logs. Everything was done by hand, we had good tools at this time, keeping them clean and sharp made all the difference.

It had warmed up considerably, our clothes were wool and buckskin. We also wore linen underneath to stop chafing. We decided just to ware the linen because it was getting so warm in the sun, this wouldn't happen back at our village. It would make a heck of a scandal seeing men working in there underclothes. We laughed a lot seeing ourselves working in underclothes. We were also very fortunate to be able to afford linen.

We took a day off to relax and look at our handiwork, it was hard to believe everything went so well. I decided that afternoon I would go and look for the Indians to trade with. I would take a few knives, hatchets and a few pans just enough to let them know what I had to trade. The next morning I was on My Way, Chuck and Chum wished me good luck. I had my skinning knife plus what I called my fighting knife on my left shoulder. I also made sure I had flint for starting a fire and took the dried food we had prepared back home. I would not have to start a fire to cook only if I wanted to.

I had always ridden bareback, my filly was not used to having something hang on her backside. Took some time for me to settle her down. She was quite frisky, she finally settled down when she realize I would still be on her back. I didn't realize that I had not use reins in a long time, she sensed my knee pressure would turn stop run like heck depending on my position. This had been natural for both. Everyday woodworking she would look for me if I didn't show up right away. If I didn't acknowledge her, she would give me a nudge with her nose.

So off I went, Chum thought about coming with me but I said I will be back in four or five days. Chuck and Chum would finish up some of the fine-tuning on the building and had time would build a lean to for the horses and other outside things.

I travelled leisurely enjoying the land and nature, stirring up a lot of grouse and seeing quite a few deer. The first day I stopped as it got dark and found a good spot to rest and let my filly feed. We were staying close to the stream as we travelled. I knew that a village would be near water, the second day went by about the same, I was enjoying the country. It seemed a little drier than I was used to. Nights had been pleasant I enjoyed the night sound, I had excellent night vision. I had discovered this while hunting with a few of the villagers. They had a hard time seeing to get out of the woods after dark. They would just follow me and do a lot of stumbling even then. I found later on they would not hunt with Chum and me because of this. Chum also had good night vision. We would hunt till after dark and found most animals moved early or just before dark this is when we had our best luck.

The next day travelled all morning still not seeing any sign of Indians or a village. Late afternoon I spotted a doe feeding. There were other deer also but she was real close. I decided what the heck, I would enjoy a good chunk of deer roasted over a fire. I took careful aim and shot the deer the neck, she dropped right there. I went and cut her throat to drain out the blood and then started to gut her out. My filly got quite fidgety, I ignored her and kept on the chore of gutting the doe. I should have paid better attention to my filly, I was rapped aside the head and went out cold. When I came to I was trussed up and laying on the back of my filly with the doe. I knew if they had tried to ride my filly she would have done her best to buck them off. She would not let any strangers get on and stay on her back. They probably had a hard time getting near her. I believe they used me to calm her down, I found out later she had kept coming over to me even though I was still out cold, this is when they loaded me and the deer on my filly. They only had three horses and there were six of them, three of the Indian just ran alongside the horses. I spent the night on the ground with the doe. The next morning I was loaded up again with the doe. It was evening before we got to the village. By that time it was almost dark. They just dumped me in the teepee and left. I don't know why but I was the only one in the tepee. They had taking my fighting knife and my outside belt with my gutting and skinning knife along with all the things I carried my rifle flint etc.

They had not taken any of my clothes off soon be known to them, I had a small knife in my underclothes.. When I had gone to the bath house in the city my knives were stolen, so this knife was hid in my clothes. I wiggled enough to get the knife out of my underclothes. I waited until I could hear no more noise from the outside, this is when I cut myself loose. I was going to cut a hole in the tepee and decided against it. That would be a dead giveaway of where I was going and where I went. Next thing I did I took off my shoes which were more or less heavy moccasins. Being barefoot I could be a lot quieter, then I went to the flap on the tepee to look out. There was a guard sitting there any seem to wake for a few seconds but as I watched he dosed back off again.

I then came up with the idea of going to hide where they dumped refuse also did all the defecating etc.. I knew if I was to escape, I would have to have my filly. Being very careful, I eased out of the tepee by the guard. He just seemed to be snoring lightly as I went by. I knew other refuse place would be on the other side of the village away from the two trails coming in. Just as I got to the fire pit, someone was coming out of latrine area. Then I dropped down next to the pit almost laying down not to be seen. I recognize it as a woman coming up out of the latrine area. As she went into the tepee I stayed quiet for a little while longer. I then came up with the bright idea, Filled my shoes with fire ashes from the pit, then proceeded to the refuse area. Just on the other side there was a knoll with a lot of grass overlooking the village. From this knoll I would be able to see the goings on in the village the next morning. It was one of the longest nights I believe I could ever remember. As the day broke I saw the guard get up and get something to drink. He went back to the tepee went in came out and made some type of noise to wake up the others. It wasn't long before there was quite commotion. Two or more Braves in and out of the tepee this started a search for my tracks. First they checked on my filly she was still in the holding area with the other horses. Next a tracker went around the tepee in ever larger circles looking for my tracks. This is when I was glad I had not cut my way out of the tepee. That would've been a giveaway of exactly where I'd went. I wasn't sure what would be my next move but decided to wait and see if everything, calmed down some. Next thing that happened was the main tracker got two others to start circling the village. I watched as they circled the village. I just laid down watching without making any movement. This way wouldn't give myself away and it would be awfully hard to see me laying in the high grass. In a short while I heard the tracker come by and pass very close fortunately didn't see me.

There was a lot of excitement and commotion that morning. Late morning the chief and two Braves started out on horses the others followed on foot. I could see the trackers head for the stream and started looking for tracks along the stream they knew I would need water, but could get by without food, but not water.

Later when everything calm down, I decided to make my move. The women working at different chores. I was very careful to sneak around into the wind and be on the side hill. It took me a good hour or more. When I got partway down the hill I proceeded to moan deep down as much as I could. This brought the attention of all the woman in the camp. I threw the ashes in the air and stepped through the dust taking long strides but not running. I went up and touched one of the older Indian woman on the arm. Then headed over to the eating area. I was parched not having any water for so long. I drink my fill and then ate some of the leftovers. This is when I put my shoes back on. Everyone in the camp saw me so it would not make any difference if I had my shoes on or not.

I had also watched the Braves when they left, no one could stay on my filly so they just took her long riderless. She was willing to follow the other horses. I knew without my horse I would have a hard time getting back to our encampment. Decided to try to make

A Past Life: As Told By Brave Hawk

peace with the men and the chief when they came back. I waited behind a large tree

They would come back on that well used trail. As the chief and the other Braves came riding into the view, I waited until they were about 30 feet or so then stepped out raising my hand in a peace sign. One of the Braves knocked an arrow to his bow. I thought for sure I had had it. Could hear behind me the other older woman and others were hollering not to shoot. The way I had appeared to them was something they had never experienced and figured I must have a lot of spirit protection. The chief then put his hand on the brave and he lowered the bow. The chief then slid off his horse and came right up to me and put his hand on my shoulder. This is when I was sure I was going to be all right.

Was welcomed into the tribe. The village wasn't overly large, about 20 to 30 people. One older boy about 12 a few small children and one baby. What surprised me was there were no dogs in this village. I was told by older men who had met with a lot of Indian tribes that there were always numerous dogs in each village. I was very fortunate because if there had been dogs they would probably have betrayed me.

That evening they put on the feast, it was the doe that I had killed. They also grew different vegetables, and dried berries and other foods I could not identify, one was squash and pumpkin.

Next day all my belongings were returned. My filly was glad to see me and I her. I was surprised they only had three horses. The chief is the only one that seemed to know how to handle his horse. The other two Braves were having a hard time but got along quite well.

That evening they had a big get-together and big feed I met all the Braves and their Shaman. He was the chief's father, I believe he and the chief thought I had pulled off some kind of shenanigan, but didn't know what or how. I knew I would have to make up some kind of fairytale. Everyone was anxious to find out how I got out of the tepee and where I was most of the next day. The three main trackers knew I had left no tracks around the village. They had not picked up any tracks even downstream from the stream that went by the village.

Through sign language they conveyed to me the question of where I was hiding. This is when I decided to fabricate how I had gotten away. I had been informed even before I left on our adventure, that the Indians were spiritual and also a little superstitious. I began by telling them when I came to in the tepee I asked my spirits to help me. And then just concentrated on that, the next thing I knew the spirit came through the top of the tepee and cut me loose and took me out the top of the tepee. Then I floated over the top of the village. I proceeded to tell him what was going on in the village, how everyone got really excited and went in and out of the tepee. The next thing I said that trackers went around the tepee three times, then two went one way around the village the other went the other way. Spirit held me up for a long time then drop me down in a puff and I floated down to touch the older woman, to let the woman and children know I was there.

Then went over to the eating place and proceeded to get something to eat and drink I was really dry not drinking for almost two days. This is when the woman said I didn't make any tracks at all until I had drank and had something to eat. I was glad I'd put my shoes back on this is the tracks I was leaving so it made it look as though I went from semi spirit to solid again.

I don't believe the old Shaman and chief really believed my story. But they had no way of refuting it. Even the trackers were spellbound. I later found out how good all the trackers were at really tracking. I thought I was real good. I would be just an amateur compared to them.

I asked about not seeing any dogs around. I had been told to expect to see quite a few dogs in most villages. This was another

A Past Life: as told by Brave Hawk

coincidence that allowed me to pull off my escape from the tepee. The dogs would have more than likely given me away. They related to be a very sad story, two of the dogs had come down with rabies they had bitten one older child two of smaller children and one of the woman. They had killed all the dogs for fear they also may have had rabies. The loss for the tribe because of the rabies was very painful. One was a chief's wife and child. One thing I was thankful for they had not stripped my clothes off, they would have found my small knife and I would not have been able to get free.

The next day I roamed around the village and met everyone. At first I didn't know what was going on they seem to be having some kind of conference. Later I found they wanted to adopt me into the tribe. I was very attracted to the chiefs sister. I thought she was his wife she was staying in the same tepee as the chief and his mother. I couldn't believe I was so attracted to this girl. I found out later that the Chiefs mother wanted to adopt me. The chief could see that his sister was very attracted to me and me to her. This is when he told his mother if she adopted me I would be a brother and I would not be able to marry her daughter. Chiefs mother then said I would gain a son anyway if they married.

The older woman that I had touched on the arm when I came and made my debut from the spirit world. Had Lost an older son. She wanted to adopt me in the worse way. She did have a 12-year-old son but would welcome me as her older son. It took quite a while for them to conveyed their intentions to me. Once I knew what was wanted. I was elated I couldn't hide my exuberance. They got a big kick out of me when I went into my cartwheels and jumps etc. The Braves never showed much emotion, but they all had good laugh at my antics. This is the first time they released the stolid features and smiled and laughed.

I was enjoying the village and the few small children. I got into their games, I would pick one up and twirl him or her and set them down At the other end 0f the Village. They wanted me to race them from one end of the village to the other. Once I set them down they would run like heck . I would run behind and let them win. The woman were amazed at my playing with the children this way. With a smaller toddlers I would get on my hands and knees to race them. They just ran in any direction not always toward the finish line. They had other games also one was rolling hoops and shooting arrows threw the hoops, quite a challenge.

I had never grown up around many small children was a lot of fun for me. The Chiefs sister joined me and I found she was very quick and fast. She would deliberately bump me and knock me off stride then laugh like heck. I couldn't get over how much I was enjoying this village. The men and the boys would join in with their bows . I had never tried a bow before, they got me to try. I didn't do very well. I could see it took a lot of practice to be as good as the men were They were exceptionally good. I then decided that I would become a darn good Bowman. I would make a bow and do a lot of practicing. Shooting a rifle gave some advantage to learning to shoot well with a bow. I was determined to learn at a later date.

Within a couple of days they had adoption ceremony. I asked where I could be alone to bathe. Through a lot of hand signals the Chiefs mother and daughter and my adopted to be mother. They told me there was a pool just upstream that was perfect for bathing. I then called my filly by whistling to her. She came on a trot, she had just jumped right over their enclosure and came to me. And she nuzzled me to let me know she was there. They were amazed at the way that she had came at my whistle.

They gave me some kind of soap , they also gave me some kind of herb that smelled real good. I mounted my filly and offered Running Deer a ride. She turned me down so I headed upstream. I had just learned her name that day. She followed me on the run. Found the spot disrobed down to my linen underwear. When in the pool I ducked down to get my head wet. I looked at the bank and Running Deer was gathering up my clothes, I didn't know what she

A Past Life: As Told By Brave Hawk

had planned. It was to wash my clothes in the pool. She was sorting my clothes out and she came across my small knife in my under belt. Her eyes got real big as she looked at me. I just shrugged my shoulders, and she doubled over laughing. Now I thought everybody would know how I got loose from the rawhide bindings. Then she tapped her mouth letting me know that she wouldn't say anything. This let me know that my secret was safe with her. That was one heck of a relief for me. I knew later on I would tell her what I had done and how lucky I was. One tracker had came within 150 feet of where I was hiding. He was concentrating on the ground for tracks and not so much on the landscape.

I knew I had to get back to the log place and let them know I was all right. I didn't want them to come looking for me, the Indians here weren't very friendly toward white men. This is when I told them I would be back. I left a lot of my belongings in my mother's to be tepee. This showed them I would return I just took some food and water in and even left my rifle.

When it was time to leave the chief advised me that there was another tribe downstream a few miles. They knew about me now because one of their Braves was here visiting. He had left right after I had related how I had escaped. She told me they might try something to enhance the power of their tribe. The shaman was a instigator for trouble. Leaving in the later morning everyone wished me well and to return. That first night in high spirits and enjoying the country this time if my filly made a racket I would be prepared.

On my way early next morning, about mid-morning found three Braves following me. This is not a good sign for me. They would have given me the peace sign if their intentions were peaceful. This is when I kept my filly to the left of the well-used trail. This would give me advantage of being right-handed. Could see that the one brave had his, Tomahawk in his right hand .They were out of my sight , Just as I topped the sharp rise this is when the Brave made his move. I heard him gooses his horse I then turned my filly slightly sideways. He wasn't expecting me to be right there. He had his Tomahawk raised but his horse moved to his right to avoid my filly. Then my action was to make a hard slash to his throat as his horse tried to avoid mine. This had gave me advantage over him. I had slicing his throat from ear to ear. I then goosed my filly and turned her to face the other two as they came up over the rise. I then made a slashing motion with my knife. This is when the other brave fell off his horse. Their eyes got very large could see that one was a lot older than the other. Both thought I had cut the Braves throat when I had made the slashing motion from a distance. The old shaman had heard about my escape and thought he could make some prestige for his tribe if he could do me in. They were going to load the brave and bring him back to their village. I was angry enough I made them bury him right there. They had a hard time digging a grave but I would not let up until it was done.

Without the Chiefs warning I probably wouldn't have been prepared. This is when I decided to push my filly a little faster. I arrived quite early on the third day. Chuck and Chum were getting quite worried. Being gone a week or better was upsetting. So them seeing me come in made for a very happy get-together. They had just made breakfast so all enjoyed breakfast.

Then proceeded to tell about what had happened and how I escaped. They got a big kick out of this. But I also stated how lucky I was. I then told them I was going back to the village with some of our trade goods. We didn't bring an awful a lot of goods on our first trip we needed our tools more so. Some of the building tools were left for future use. So going back would be a lot lighter, the to wheel carts would be empty.

We decided to leave one of the draft horses with me. I would use him as a my pack horse. We had brought nice hatchets pots and frying pan. Being in the village I could see these would be well welcome. We finish up some of the things we wanted to do to seal

A Past Life: As Told by Brave Hawk

up our openings. We left no food or anything that would attract any animal by the odors. We had done all our cooking outside having no chimney as yet. We had built a lien-to in case of rain so that we could cook without getting wet. This was used for fodder for some of the horses. Horses didn't have much of a problem. They seem to do very well on the grasses that abounded. The grasses must been very nutritional because they did well.

Our trip had gone quite well for the first time. On the way back Chuck and Chum said they would improve on the route to find the easiest way. They also are going to find a man or a couple of men to run the trading post. Chum told me aunt Sue might make the trip after things were set up and well-established. I was sure Chuck would be back. Maybe in future runs, Chuck just wanted to make sure we didn't get into any trouble. He knew the trip could be made without any major hardships. The two wheeled cards worked out much better than wagon still carried a good load. The only thing was to make sure they were balanced right.

We said our goodbyes and proceeded on our way. Took my time back wasn't about to shoot another deer! The attention I would receive would be very welcome. So I lazily rode, enjoying the country. Couple of days riding found the village that the old shaman and young Indian that I had killed came from. Rode into the village and they were surprised that I was stopping, because of what the old shaman had tried to do. I ignored the men got off my filly. Then unpacked a few of the pots and pans knives and I gave them to the oldest Indian woman there. Then packed up and left for my village. I knew everyone would be envious of her. I knew the Braves love those knives that I had given her. Everyone just stared at me. I believe now that they were afraid I would pull out my knife and cut someone's throat.

Another day or so and I rode into the village, all were very glad to see me and me them. Even the kids gave me a big welcome, they weren't sure if I would be back. I never felt more like home here. That evening ahead of the meal was trying hard to learn the language. They would burst out with laughter at some of my pronunciations.

The next day they went out hunting for fresh game. They included me in this hunt . This is when I found how good the trackers were. They would see things I was completely overlooking. Their best tracker took a liking to me and was going out of his way to teach me some of his techniques. I was flabbergasted at the things he could see. I knew I would never be as good as he was. But would do better than a lot because of his teachings. About midday and two deer were killed. We then headed back to the village. I found the trackers when tracking were barefoot. They didn't put on their moccasins until the hunt was over.

The pots and pans knives and hatches were well received. I had not asked for anything in trade. Most didn't know how to handle this, they were great traders and something was always expected in return. So I conveyed to them this was my gift to them for adopting me. I gave the best hatchet and knife to the chief.

I had been staying with the chief his mother and sister. We had moved my belongings into my soon-to-be adopted mothers tepee with her younger son. We had got along real well before I left so he welcomed me. They insisted I take the best spot in the tepee.

Next thing was I had to be bathed, I thought the men would do the bathing. When I got to the pool all the woman were there. I just striped down to my underwear made sure my small knife had been left back at the tepee just in case they were going to wash my clothes again.

Some other woman are already in the pool SO I WENT INTO THE POOL AND THEY ducked me under and pulled my underwear off before I realized what was going on. I received the most thorough scrubbing of my life.

A Past Life: as told by Brave Hawk

At first I was going to give them a tussle but thought this is part of their ceremony so just relax never being naked with a bunch of woman had turned me red without the scrubbing.

After relaxing I enjoyed the bath. I found it very invigorating. The evening was spent with a lot of dancing and drumming. Before long I was gathered up and brought before the shaman and my mother to be. After some chanting and it seem like blessings, took my right arm and made a small cut and did the same on my adopted mothers right arm. Cut was at the wrist, then we put our hands on each others arm and the blood was to mix and make us mother and son. The shaman then put something on each wound, he did some more chanting then acknowledge we were now mother and son. A lot of hooping and yelling, this is when they got me up to dance with them. It was a wonderful night, everyone had a real good time. Also the food was excellent, woman did their best effort to make everything pleasant and tasty, and they did a real good job. The next morning everyone slept in, including myself we had tired ourselves out dancing most of the night.

A few days later the woman gathered their baskets to go berry picking and forging for herbs and vegetables. They also had a garden that was well cared for. They found a big patch of berries and a Valley not too far from the village. My new brother came with us only because I was going along. I would pick berries and would then dumped what I picked into my mothers or one of the older woman's basket. They would just laugh and shake their head.

I would sneak up and grab a handful of berries out of running dears basket. She would grab the basket chase me off.

I grabbed a handful, she picked up a stick to chased me I then ran and got behind my adopted mother. Stood with her arms crossed daring Running Dear to come near. When the other see my antics, made them break out with laughter and Running Deer just shook her stick at me and went back to picking berries. I could tell she was getting a big kick out of my shenanigans like the rest were.

My new brother just watched. He went up on a small rise to watch he didn't know what to make of me. He had never seen any men that picked berries with the woman. All of a sudden he yelled a warning I looked up and on a hill about hundred and fifty feet or so away was a brave and he had his bow and was proceeding to aim at me. I knew at this distance I would see the arrow if I just stepped sideways when he let loose his arrow.

I stepped to the side and had my knife out and knocked the arrow down, he had already put another arrow and had let loose the second one, I stepped left and was very fortunate to also knock that arrow down. He then left in a hurry. Some of the woman had fled to warn the village if it hadn't been for my Indian brother I don't believe I would be a alive. They didn't go into hugging so I just put my hands on his shoulders and closed my eyes and brought my head to his.

Two of the trackers showed up shortly. Then my brother showed them where the other brave that shot his arrows at me was standing I was going to go with them. They shook their heads to let me know I should go back to the village. I watched them as they went over to where the brave was standing, when he shot his arrows. They took one look and were out off at a trot. I hope to have them teach me about tracking the way they did.

They didn't show up at the village till evening. They were now sure another village shaman had sent their best Bowman out to get me. It would have given the village great prestige.

When the woman and my young brother told them I had just flicked both arrows away from me, it was hard for them to believe it. I tried to tell them that they could do this also, if they were at a distance in slightly off to the side. They were still in awe of this. I hadn't thought it was such a big thing.

I was grateful for is my younger brother giving me the warning. When I explained this to them and they praised him. I could see

A Past Life: As Told by Brave Hawk

this gave him a wonderful feeling, he would come and stand by my side. I knew then if I ever had to I would forfeit my life for him.

The trackers said they knew what village the brave had come from, he had come on foot. He had been watching for a couple of days, waiting to get a chance to shoot at me. They told me they could have caught up with him but wanted to see what other village he had come from. After the woman and my brother related how I had flicked the arrows away, they were glad they had not caught him. The story he would tell would more than likely be much exaggerated.

The chief and the old shaman shook their heads then said my spirits were protecting me. No one had ever seen anyone knock an arrow out of the air. As much explanation as I gave, they would just nod and motioned that the spirits were protecting me. I now had to agree with them.

Running Dear and I were together now all the time. I had guessed her aged 16 to 18, she was not very big but was like myself very agile and fast. I finally learned how to ask the chief and his mother if I could marry Running Deer. The chief the shaman and my stepmother to be got together and talked. They agreed and also said the goods I had brought back would be good for the bride price. At the time I didn't understand this. This was accustomed that a bride price was to be paid. It would be quite a while before this would happen. I had no idea why, but being a chiefs sister they wanted to let other villages know it was going to happen. This would give them all a chance to come if they wanted.

It wasn't long before a large Indian and two Braves came into the village. He was leading two beautiful pinto ponies. He just went to the feeding area and proceeded to help himself. I got the impression he was a bully because of his size he could intimidate everyone around him. The kids all seem to disappear when he showed up.

My adopted mother and bride-to-be wanted me to leave. Apparently they knew why he had come. A couple of days past I could tell he was watching me all the time. The evening was progressing and everyone seemed to be on edge . This Guy wasn't very well-liked and no one went near him if they didn't have to.

That evening he parked himself fairly close to the food. As I walked by he stuck his Tomahawk out and motioned for me to bring him something from the food rack. I turned and spit on him. Now all hell broke loose, he came at me with both his Tomahawk. My adopted mother and the other woman stepped in and put up a barrier between me and him. He backed off with a mean grin on his face. My mother then insisted I go back to our tepee. My brother came on the run, I believe he would have taken on the Indian in my defense. When I got back to the tepee my things were all packed and she wanted me to leave. She said this is why that brave showed up, he wanted to pick a fight with me.

My Indian brother told me this brave had killed quite a few men in challenges. After a couple of days of watching me he figured I was an easy target.

The chief came then told me that he had come to him with this challenge. What I had done was one of the worst insults you could muster to insult another brave. The only recourse was a fighting challenge. If I decline his challenge I would have to leave. My bride-to-be would more than likely be his. I wasn't about to Leave and Not Accept the Challenge.

My bride-to-be came and told me she would leave with me right away. This is when I said no way was I going to leave like a coward.

Another couple of days past my mother insisted I stay away from the village. My bride-to-be got me to go fishing upstream with her. I realize that she just wanted to keep me out of the village and his sight. She tried to talk me into leaving but I said no I wasn't

A PAST LIFE: AS TOLD BY BRAVE HAWK

going. I was pretty good at spearing fish with my knife. We would start a fire and roasts the fish. My bride-to-be knew all about herbs to enhance the taste.

That night I tried to get into her bedding with her she just laughed and shook her head and pointed to my bedding. The next morning one of the trackers came and told me it was time to go back to the village. I asked him what I was supposed to do. I was glad I asked. I had no idea how I was supposed to act. He then drew a circle about 30 foot or so, then showed me what would happen. I was to stand on one edge of the circle and when ready step in. Then my challenger would step in and the fight would begin. This is when he said that it was a fight to the death. If either tried to leave the circle, the Braves would push them back in. At least now I knew the rules. This brave liked me I could tell he was worried. One of the small kids I played with was his I didn't realize till later on that the braves all just put on the Stoic front when they were worried. Most would not play with the kids like I did. I believe he was appreciated of my doing so. Some of the Braves including him had started to clown around with the little ones as I did.

Back we went into the village. We had walked not using horses and everyone in the village was very somber. I didn't know it at the time but no one thought I had a chance against this Indian. My mother brought me a light meal, my bride-to-be disappeared.

I then went to see the shaman and ask him for his blessings. He gave me a big smile and nodded and made a few chants. Next I went to see the chief, he gave me his best stone tomahawk. Then put both hands on my shoulder he also gave me a big smile.

A couple of days and Early afternoon everything was ready, this circle was drawn. I could see there were quite a few other Braves that I hadn't seen before. They were there to see what was going on and to keep anyone in the circle. The two that had came with the big Indian were also there. When I was ready I was to step into the circle tomahawk in one hand my knife in the other. I stepped into the circle right off, had the Chiefs tomahawk in my left hand my fighting knife in my right.

The circle was in a place where all the villagers could watch from a Hill. I was watching the Indian I was to fight, what I observed before, he seemed a little on the clumsy side. He looked over at me and stepped into the circle raising his Tomahawk's and gave a hell of a yell. This is when I made three large running steps leaping in the air catching his tomahawk with my left hand which held the Chiefs tomahawk. Twisting at the same time I drove my knife down into his neck and chest, landing on my feet near the edge of the circle facing him. He stood still for a very short time dropped both his tomahawk and put his hands out to the two braves that had came with him, they turned their backs and walked away. There wasn't any movement except for the two braves walking away.

All the braves around the circle were stunned. They had expected me to run around the circle to try to keep out of his reach and maybe get a lick or two in before he did me in, none had expected me to survive this match. He had won every challenge he had entered. The old shaman and the chief were the only ones that new for sure I would win. Of course my mother did also.

I learned later how disgusted the Braves that came with him were with his actions, also all the other Braves that were there watching. They expected him to turn on me with his last breath an still fight. Instead he had just dropped his tomahawks and went to the two braves that came with him.

When I realize he was down for good, I did not know what I was supposed to do. I turned my knife and Tomahawk around and went over and handed them to the chief. He took them and went over and wiped both sides of the knife and tomahawk on the brave.

The villagers on the hill had just settled down to watch and didn't realize it was all over. Most didn't see any of the action they all thought I would try running around in the circle to tire my

A Past Life: as told by Brave Hawk

opponent out. All I could think of was thanking Chuck for his instructions about fighting. One main rule was always to make the first move if possible. Chuck had said this usually was the most telling blow. The chief then came back and handed me my knife and tomahawk.

Everyone was stunned, the fight lasted less than a minute and a half at the most. The old Shaman that I asked to bless me was there also. The chief had a slight grin on his face. When I looked at the old shaman he just gave me a nod. The villagers on the hill were still waiting to see the action, they couldn't believe it was over. They had not really settled down to watch so missed all of the action.

My Indian mother had watched and she had told all that she knew her son would win because the spirit favoured him. How else would I have flicked two arrows out of the air that were meant to kill me. I was learning how much prestige and bravery meant to the Indians. I also realize how much there's stories were exaggerated. I still tried to tell about knocking arrows aside. They just nodded and grinned.

I found that the word from the other Braves that came, believed I couldn't be killed by an arrow. My spirits were too strong. I didn't realize but the brave that had shot at me was also among the large group of strange Indians. He was the one that was telling all the other Indians that I had deflected his arrows back at him and he was very fortunate to escape.

That evening there was a celebration by my village. Others had brought t fish meat and herbs, food goods of all kinds. They had planned on celebrating on my passage to the spirit world. By my not passing was a better reason to have the feast.

When I walked through the village, strange Indians that I hadn't seen before just stared at me when I passed by. They couldn't believe how small I was compared to the brave I had just done in. It made me quite uncomfortable, I tried to find a spot out-of-the-way hoping no one would notice me. Just didn't like this attention. I ended up going to the Chiefs teepee and I was welcomed by my Indian chief and mother. I was waiting for things to calm down.

My mother came into the teepee and joined us. I then asked where my Indian maid was the last few days. My mother then told me my Indian maid had left the village for one of her favorite spots. She had told my Indian mother that she would be there. It was a special spot she was the only one that knew that went there. It was like a small grotto. I didn't realize she had gone there two days before the fight was to take place. Later I found out she had fasted for three days. This is for my success in this fight, she had told my Indian mother but no one else. Running Deer's mother and my mother were the only two who knew where the spot was. My Indian mother went to get her but she was already on her way back to the village. She had raised her hand up and told my Indian mother she knew I had won, it came in a vision while she was fasting. It was obvious to my Indian mother when she met my Indian maid she had a big smile and nodded. Running Deer went to the stream to bathe before entering the village, and the teepee.

The shaman told he had seen the fight in a vision and knew of the outcome also the chief knew. His vision was not to be known until after the fight. My Indian mother had watched and told all the villagers she wasn't worried I would come out the winner. My spirits were so much stronger than this other brave that he didn't stand a chance.

The next day the Braves that came with my challenger brought the ponies and his horse and all his belongings to the teepee. They made sure I knew they had brought them and all his belongings. I accepted, they just gave a nod and left. Found out later that this Indian had killed six or eight in a similar challenge. The chief said there won't be too many that would challenge me now.

The feast started next day all kinds of things games, Bow shooting and other Indian games were going on before the big feed.

A Past Life: as told by Brave Hawk

They had running as one of the games. The woman and girls could enter. The Indian woman had made a type of woven belt for the winner of the running. I found out my Indian maid had won by a long shot all the running contest she had entered. After a kind of the elimination of all the slower runners, the best were to run. I asked if it was okay to enter the contest all just nodded. I knew back in my own village I had won also by a long shot. There was not much competition for me.

The race was quite long and could be observed for a mile or more. We started out everyone ran real hard at first. Running Deer and myself lag back for a while. Then my Indian maid took the lead, I was right at her side, she stepped up the pace. We left everyone behind, as we came to the last turn she was running the outside of the turn and I tripped her, she stumbled I made a beeline for the finish. Stopping about 30 feet from the finish line. She was only one step behind me she also stopped I could see she was upset by my actions. We both just stood there, then the shaman came over and handed me this belt, figured I would have crossed the finish line first. I then took the belt and put it around my maids shoulders. She was surprised at this, I tried to get her to cross the finish line ahead of me. She refused and turned sideways, this is when I grabbed her around the waist picked her up from behind and carried her almost over my head and set her down on the other side of the finish line. I then grabbed her hand and walked with her for the next few paces. This is when the woman watching made some kind of noise with her hand over their mouth which was very loud. Thought I had done something wrong again. My Indian maid then gave me a big smile and squeeze my hand then I realize this was meant as a sign of high approval. I knew if I had not tripped her she more than likely would've won by at least one pace. She was the only one that had ever given me any running competition and really could have beaten me. She also wasn't very big I had had no problem picking her up.

Really didn't know all of things they had for the feast but everything was delicious, to my taste anyway.

After a few days when things calmed down, I got to thinking about the log building that we constructed. I was wondering how it fared in my absence. Asking some of the Braves and trackers if they wanted to go and see what had brought me out West to their territory. The chief decided to come also. The next day we left and travelled quite fast. Surprised me how quick we got to the building. Everything looked fine there were also two men there that Chum and already hired. One name was Judd, he seemed to be the one in charge. He then told us that Chum would be back with supplies to trade. We then headed back. We had killed a number of grouse and had a good feed. Most of the Braves were good enough shots with a bow to knock these grouse out of the air. My brother being quite young was still an excellent shot with a bow, I sure could learn from him. After a leisurely ride we returned to the village.

I asked the chief about the horses I had won in the challenge fight if they were enough for the bride price. He just grinned and said that the tools and pots and pans were accepted as a bride price, the horses were mine. I then gave the pinto pony to my Indian maid. One of the others was given to my brother. I knew now that I couldn't just give the other horse away. I knew the best tracker liked me and I liked him very much, he would have liked the horse the brave I killed had been riding. Trying to think of something I could ask in trade for the horse. He did have bows and arrows and other things I asked for but this didn't seem appropriate. Approaching him and his teepee with the horse, I squatted down in a sitting position noting I wanted to trade the horse. At first he thought I wanted his woman. Very embarrassing for me I should have sent some one first to let my intention be known. I got the message across that I wanted a bow and arrows also wanted him to teach me some of his tracking skills. He finally understood what I wanted. He hemmed and hawed I didn't think he was going to trade. Me not knowing this was one way of showing that his values were equal to mine. When he seen the disappointment look on my face he then smiled and agreed to trade. Was surprised when he agreed, I had jumped up and did a little dance. He and his woman doubled over with laughter. My antics were not very Indian like, even though well-received. I was very glad he had accepted.

The very next day he came and got me for foraging hunt. I was totally amazed at the things he could see. He would point things out and try to explain their meaning. Sometimes I knew, other times I couldn't quite see what he was seeing .He sent l Little Arrow ahead of us and had me start tracking him. Didn't have to much trouble at first, then the earth became hard pact and a lot of rock ledges. Lost his tract Gonacheaw then said his track is there. He then made me bend over and look closer. I was amazed could now see an outline glow of his foot. Gonacheaw could do this on a run. I now could do it but at a walk. All of a sudden the tracks disappeared. Gonacheaw said Little Arrow is now hiding his tracts .Really concentrate you will see them again. After a few minutes was able to pick them up again. Gonacheaw told me Little Arrow and I were the only ones he knew could do this, he then told me he would teach me to see my back trail and also front trail also. A few day's later he again said he knew was able to see many miles ahead and back of me. Gonacheaw had sent Little Arrow about five miles out on one of the trails. Little Arrow was to act like he was to ambush me. Gonacheaw told me to concentrate. It came to me shortly. Told gonacheaw knew were he was and told him where I was seeing Little Arrow. He smiled and nodded. We took off on the run to approach Little Arrow, he knew I had located him. We three were very pleased that it had gone so fast and well. Gonacheaw said you have it now can do this also on your back trail.

Back East Chum and I were considered excellent trackers. But we were both novices compared to him and the other trackers of the tribe. I made up my mind someday I would tell him how I had eluded him and the other trackers. My tracks coming out of the tent had been covered up by everyone going in and out of the tepee. They didn't treat trespassers very well at that time. I would more than likely have been killed. No dogs and my hidden knife were the things that made very fortunate circumstances that aided my escape.

My Bride had shared the tepee with the chief, her brother, his wife and the old shaman who was the chief's grandfather. The shaman also had a small tepee of his own. He used this most of the time for ceremonies etc.

Getting ready for my wedding, I was in for another scrubbing by the woman. Except this time my Bride to be would not be with them. She and her mother were preparing for the ceremony. I didn't actually know what I was supposed to do. My Indian mother moved out with my Indian brother, this was temporary. I found that my bride knew more about lovemaking than I did, we were both virgins. I was quite clumsy. We giggled and laugh and after a while everything went smoothly. We thoroughly enjoyed one another. We stayed in the tepee for the next few days. The third day we emerged and we headed up to the pool and bathed then enjoyed each other. We could swim in the pool but it wasn't very large. Still we enjoyed it. I couldn't believe how fortunate and happy I was at this time.

We decided to take a trip, she had a favorite place that was supposedly sacred. Not many went there because of the spirits that were there. At the time I didn't believe in spirits so was more than willing to go. We loaded our ponies and started out, the first day we travelled then made a camp early. We had stopped made love a few times. The next day Running Deer said we would be passing another village and after that it was only a day away. Again we stopped early afternoon my bride went foraging for I didn't know what. She had seen something she wanted for supper. I then proceeded set up our lean-to. Our lean-to was a Treated Buffalo Hide, it was waterproof and made a good windbreak also

As I was setting this lean to up, I heard some sound and my filly also whinnied. Six Braves came striding toward me, all had Tomahawks in their hands. They hollered at me and pointed at the lean to. My bride heard the commotion and came on the run. They knew her as the chiefs sister, they still didn't look very happy with my being there. Running Deer squatted down in front of them, to explain who I was and what we were doing. I went over and

A Past Life: as told by Brave Hawk

squatted next to her, I wasn't supposed to do this so she just gave me a hell of a shove and I kind of toppled over. This seems to be the funniest thing that they'd ever seen. All of them doubled over with laughter one was rolling on the ground roaring. When things subsided they were still breaking into laughter when looking at me. My bride finally told them I was the one who had fought the large brave who came into our village. They were off hunting when the fight took place. So they miss being there, but had heard about it afterward. They were glad that He was the one that lost the fight. They also had heard all about it, and it was very exaggerated by the storyteller. They were amazed at my sise had thought me to be a big man, then wanted to see the scars that he had inflicted on me. I understood but knew he had not wounded me in any way. Running Deer knew about the scars the bear had inflicted on my arm and chest. She then turned me around and proceeded to take my shirt off tapping my mouth with her fingers. In other words shut up and let her do the talking. All the Braves had to touch the scars, they didn't understand how I had healed so quickly. Running Deer told them that the spirits took care of that. They also had heard about me knocking arrows out of the air before they could harm me. They then insisted we come into their village for a feast. Again in our honor. I soon found out the brave I killed had killed two of their young Braves in a similar fight. They were more than happy to see him gone. I couldn't believe the meat they had, they had killed to Buffalo so there was much elation and partying. This is the first time I had been asked by any Indian if I had any whiskey. He even knew what the name was. I gave the sign that is no good, he just laughed.

Found out later he went through our belongings looking for whiskey. When I found out I was very upset. Running Deer, calmed me down, he took nothing just wanted whiskey. Apparently some trapper had given him whiskey and he wanted more. I never drank and didn't care for any alcohol drink, except for a small glass of wine at a meal and didn't miss that. I was finding out that the Indians had a lot of different rules. If our belongings had been in a tepee he would not have touched anything. Consequences from the tribe would have been severe.

I met their chief and was invited to stay in his tepee with his wife and children. Running Deer knew how to turn down his offer without offending him and his wife. There shaman was a very old man. He lived by himself in a small tepee, he had asked the chief to tell me he wanted to see me. The chief was surprised usually someone searched him out. Not him asking for someone. I was thrilled to meet with the old man. I also asked if Running Deer could a company me as interpreter. He was just sitting inside of the small tepee the sides were lifted for the summer. Running Deer had instructed me ahead of time how I was supposed to act and sit. He had lit some kind of herb I believe it was sage. I sat in front of him and he closed his eyes and went into a chant. When he opened his eyes he then fanned smoke over Running Deer and Myself. He then told me I would be in a battle and would be wounded and would survive and also my chief and I would become the best of friends also with the trackers. At the time I wasn't much into the spiritual thing took this as a lot of hooey. He also told me I would have some sadness but would recover with time. Running Deer then asked if we could use the holy place as a honeymoon spot. He readily agreed and gave his blessings.

After a couple of days of feasting and dancing we loaded up our horses and headed out to the holy place. Less than a day's leisurely ride we came on two streams and Lake. I believe was one of the most beautiful places I had ever witnessed. I could see why they consider it holy. Running Deer told me, no one came only on special invitation as a guest. Mostly shamans use this.

We decided to fish caught trout for supper and set up our camp. For five days of really enjoying the fishing swimming and just general loafing. Another older Indian showed up he wasn't very happy about seeing us there especially a white man. Running Deer approach him explaining we had blessing from the old shaman.

A Past Life: as told by Brave Hawk

She also told him why I was now a part of the tribe. His attitude change and welcomed us he said he would leave and come back at a later time. We insist he stay with us for the evening meal we told him we were planning on leaving in the morning anyway. He also told us that he knew he was going to meet me but didn't think it would be here. His meditation showed him the man that had done that Indian that had killed so many of the younger Braves, was spiritually protected. He asked about the Indian that had shot arrows at me if it was spirits that had defected the arrows. I didn't want to lie to him was about to answer with the truth when my bride spoke up. She said she was there and it and it was definitely my spirits who had deflected the arrows. She said she had witnessed the whole episode. This satisfied him he gave me a nod and reached over to touch me. I wanted to giggle but didn't dare. The evening went quite well, he set up his lean-to not to far from us. He told us he would start his fast for five or six days no food or water, after him telling us he knew he would meet us but had thought it at a later date. He did some chanting and meditation that evening, he came back to us, we were cuddled up next small fire. He then repeated what the old shaman had told me about getting wounded. He also told me he knew how but was forbidden to tell me but I would be just fine. Next morning I was going to get the shaman for breakfast with us. Running Deer shook her head and told me he had started his fast and it was not a good time to disturb him.

We started out I had thought we would take the same trail by. Running Deer said no we will go another route she wanted to miss the other village and get back to ours. If we went by their village they would insist we stop again, she didn't want to insult them by not accepting. This didn't hurt my feelings either. I was glad to accept her plan. Was hard to believe how well she knew all the land we were traveling. Later she said when we felt like traveling for a week or two she would show me some evil lands.

On the way back getting close to our village we met some younger Braves that were just out scouting. We had a good visit, I asked Running Deer why they acted like they knew me. She said the way you dress and the way you carry your fighting knife I was easily recognized. I could see her point. We had a good time talking, I was getting to learn the language quite well. Could not always pronounce the words but understood what was being said.

The young Braves knew we were on our honeymoon and proceeded to tease Running Deer and me. They would go through some kind of motion and gyrating their hips and laugh like heck. Back home this would never be tolerated in front of a woman. You probably would suffer some serious drubbing by some of the other men. Running Deer would hang onto my arm and laugh just as hard as they did. I realize that was part of their culture and meant no harm just good-nature d fun.

I was readily picking up their language. The harder part was getting used to their customs. When we arrived in the village everyone's got to see us. The children were after me to play with them after we settled in. My adopted mother insisted we stay with her. It was good arrangement Running Deer and she got along very well, my brother by adoption was also very happy about this arrangement.

Wasn't long before I wanted to go back to the cabin to see if Chum had made it Back with Goods for Trade. I asked the chief if he would be my partner to establish a trade culture, that he already knew much about. I would have to learn from him, felt real fortunate have him for a good friend and partner also.

The chief called the Council and had everyone who had hides to trade for goods pots pans knives hatchets or axis. We went back with a load of pelts, my pack horse and another. When we did arrive back at the building my wife was with me. Chum was there with two other men, when we rode up one of the men was startled and ran into the large buildings hollering Indians. Chum came out and welcomed me with a bear hug. Apparently I looked a lot like an Indian. We had a good time, Chum had brought different

A Past Life: as told by Brave Hawk

spices with him especially a lot of salt. This is one of the things they Indians treasure. I then introduced Chum and the two men that came with Chum to the chief and to my bride. I then told Chum we were married. He was very pleased, then introduced him directly to Running Deer. Later when alone with Chum, his first words were how lucky we both were to be married to such pretty woman. I then asked if aunt Sue was pregnant, he shook his head just shrugged his shoulders not yet. We ended up making some good trades. Our chief was a happy about the salt. We had ham that Chum had brought out for our supper also potatoes. The chief, Braves and Running Deer enjoyed the meal.

Chum told me he had hired the two men to work and improve the storehouse. I insisted no whiskey and he had not brought any. He also had made sure the two men were teetotalers. One of the mens names was Judd I didn't ask about the other. They had been there about two weeks, this is the first time anybody showed up.

Chum said he would leave the men here and go back with the Carts there was no need to cross the main river with the Carts anymore. Bringing everything over by boat now Chuck got the carpenters to build a boat that could be rowed.

I wanted to bring my bride back to meet my mom and Sue and Chuck. So asking Running Dear if she would like to go and meet my family. She readily agreed. I found my Indian language was quite good by now, learned a lot because it was all that was spoken around me.

The trip went quite well. When we got to the main river we used the boat, the horses had to swim, was afraid it might stress her pony but it didn't seem to bother There was now a small settlement on this side of the river. Chum Running Deer and myself rode up to the farm my mom was glad to see me. She had wondered if I was ever coming back. Aunt Sue was also elated. I then introduced everyone to Running Deer, telling them we had been married. Mom and Sue were absolutely delighted. We went into the house which had been expanded since I had left. Chuck was in town at the blacksmith shop and would be home for supper, which wasn't too far off. Running Deer never seeing the house before was all agog. Proceeded to show her around, we had piped water into the houses, the heat in the kitchen stove, where everything was cooked made a big impression on my bride. I told mom and Aunt Sue that the Indians ate using their fingers. They had never seen our type of knives forks and spoons. So please excuse me and Running Deer I would eat as an Indian so she wouldn't be so uncomfortable. The meal went well and Chuck was his gracious self. Told Chuck I was going into the village to see the blacksmith's I had been really fond of them and them of me.

When I showed Running Deer where we would sleep, this was in my old room mom hadn't change anything. I could tell that my bride was very apprehensive. She asked could we sleep out like we usually did. I knew it would be a tough night for her so I agreed without any argument. I had learned to love the outdoors myself, we went in and bathed before heading out to a spot in back of the house near the cemetery of my whole family. We made ourselves comfortable in our lean to and proceeded to enjoy ourselves and the outside.

The next morning we went early with the horses to my and Chum's favorite swimming hole and enjoyed a swim and a bath. Running Deer always had some real good smelling herbs, she rubbed us down with after our bath. We also washed our cloths, we then went back to the house. Mom had scrambled eggs and meat for breakfast. Running Deer did her best to follow me in my way of eating, she got the hang of the fork right away

After breakfast I wanted to go into the village and meet with the two blacksmith men who were good to me and Chum, when we worked with them. Chuck said be careful there are a few unsavory characters that had moved into the village. He was going up to the sawmill to check on some order that would be delivered in a day or two. He also said I should go up and see all the improvements

A Past Life: as told by Brave Hawk

that had been made. I told him after Running Dear and I got back we would go to the mill. Learned from mom Chuck was also the sheriff now.

Off we went to the village, didn't realize how much I now looked like an Indian. Everyone stared at us in the village heading for the blacksmith shop. As we got there someone went running into the shop, out came one of the blacksmith he recognized me and as I got off my horse he gave me one hell of a bear hug. He then hollered for his partner and out he came and did the same I then introduced them to Running Deer my new bride. One took Running Deer by the shoulders and kept nodding his head, I could tell my bride didn't know what to make of it she could see the big grin on my face and knew it was okay. She then put her hands on his shoulder and also nodded, this cracked both them up. They took off their aprons and wanted us to go into their home. I hadn't realized before they were brothers, and the younger was also married. We got to meet his wife and she was just as jolly as they were and made Running Deer and I welcome.

The man that one of the smithy was working on a project for protested. He was paying him and he wanted them to get back to work. Smithy looked at him with a big grin, spun him around and grabbed him by the seat-of-the-pants and by the caller and almost threw him back out the door. The man said he would take his business elsewhere. Smithy's reply was do that, but before you leave you had best leave coin for the work that's already been done.

We went in and sat and talked me interpreting for Running Deer. She had some kind of drink that tasted real good. We chatted for a while then it was time for us to go. We were told to come back any time for a visit or even stay over.

The Man that had been shoved out of the shop was waiting outside and had gathered a few other curious people. As we went to our ponies he made a terrible slurring remark about a half Indian and his squaw. I flash my knife off my shoulder and stepped over and told him quite politely to withdraw his words if he didn't they would be the last one's he would ever utter. My long knife was already out had drawn a little blood. His eyes were as big as saucers, he retracted in a hurry. I knew that my bride and I would never be welcome by a lot of people.

I knew how happy I was with the Indians and how well they treated me. Made up my mind when I left that would never bring my bride back again. Back home we went up to the sawmill. Running Deer was astounded to see the mill working. I showed her the waterwheel and told her Chum and I had made it.

Next day Chuck came up to me and asked what had happened in the village. I told him what had happened he smiled said he wouldn't have blame me if I had slit the blanket y-blanks throat.

Running Deer and I were ready to head back to her village. Chum said he had not got another load ready, he would be ready for a week or more. So we said our goodbyes to mom and Sue and headed back. Chum said he would get the boat and row us over which he did, then we said our goodbyes.

I carried my rifle and also carried my bow and arrow. After much coaching I was quite good with the bow but not anywhere as good as the trackers and some of others. Now being able to talk quite fluently in the Indian language, I told Running Deer I wasn't ever going back home. She just smiled and kind of shrugged her shoulders.

The chief, I and some of the others went on trading forays. We did quite well but still were in need of horses. We had found the Pawnees had a lot more than we had. They were starting to be able to kill Buffalo quite easily. They had watched the Sioux who were masters at killing Buffalo. They told us they would just ride up next to a Buffalo and were able at close range put an arrow into the ribs and sometimes hit the heart, even if they miss the heart the lungs were always struck, it wasn't long before they went down from the lung puncture.

In our trading we also planned on trading for some dogs. The village had missed having them around. I found they were very hard disciplinarians with the dogs. They were made to obey and used harsh ways of controlling them, if they couldn't control a dog in a certain length of time he became the next dog meal. I still wasn't very enthused about eating dog.

Everything seemed to be going quite well everyone seemed very contented. The Winters were not that harsh so far. They told me they had suffered the winters before they had horses. The horse let them move the village a lot easier. They also found it much easier using horses. We had six horses for the whole village when the village was moved we made a couple of trips to get everything moved. It didn't seem as though they had a lot of belongings," tepees cooking things etc. it all added up.

Running Deer and I would take time to go to the sacred place every so often. The old shaman had told us we were welcome anytime. I later found out not too many were extended this invite. The old man had a rare talent and seem to know when anyone was coming. He chose who would use this sacred place. If he said no they knew better than to disobey. If they did they didn't last long. The Braves of his tribe would find him and his life was forfeited

This became Running Deer and my favorite spot just relax and rejuvenate. The shaman always knew when we were coming and always gave us a big welcome. I was under the impression he stayed there all the time, but he didn't only when he had his visions, he then went back to the village.

Running Deer informed me she was going to have a baby, we were both really excited. Her hard exertion such as running contests she started to refrain from. She wasn't a big girl not much over 100 pounds everything seemed to go quite well, not ever complaining and keeping up with the rest of the woman. There had not been any babies born except for one that was a month or two old. We were sitting down around the fire pit and had just finished eating. The mother came by me and turned and put the baby on my lap. Never holding a baby before I was stunned didn't know what to do. My eyes were as big as saucers, when they see how I acted a lot of laughter ensued the mother just smiled and picked her baby backup. For a while any woman that went by me looked at me and broke out laughing again.

Late summer was when Running Deer was due. I hovered around her trying to anticipate her every need. She would give me a shove and tell me to go with the men they were going on a hunt on foot. She knew how much I love to be with the head tracker, I was learning a lot. I knew I would never be as good as he was. My brother had seen some deer tracks not too far from the village. She encouraged me to go with him and the tracker to see if we could have fresh deer meat for a couple of meals. We were gone much of the day when we spotted 4 or 5 deer we watched to see which way they were moving sending my brother around in front to get shot with his bow myself and the tracker separated to see if we could corral them toward my brother, we ended up with two of the deer, was still amazed how good they were with the bow. I was just beginning to shoot well with the bow. In any competition I wouldn't be able to best them. Between the three of us we carried the deer over our neck and shoulders. They insisted on carrying a deer most of the time.

We got to the village dropped the deer and all the organs by the fire pit. The woman would do the rest of the work Running Deer had went into labor while we were gone. I was not allowed into the tepees, the older woman were assisting her. Didn't realize she had been in labor shortly after we had left. Then came and got me and told me this is a woman's thing. So we all sat down for our evening meal. Most had already eaten, I was not able to eat much. They all knew something was wrong. Running Deer crossed over during the night with the baby. My mother told me and I was stunned,

A Past Life: as told by Brave Hawk

I just went outside the village and laid on the ground. I was there the rest of the night and almost all the next day. My Indian brother was there, when I came around he insisted I drink some water. I agreed then went to my filly and mounted. I knew where to go, the sacred place we had enjoyed so much. The chief told my brother to take my weapons and some of my belongings and travel food and follow me. I didn't push my filly just rode mostly at a walking pace. My brother stayed behind just out of sight. He could have rode alongside of me and I don't think I would have even known he was there. When I finally arrived at the sacred place I stripped down and waded into the lake. At this time the old shaman was there he seemed to know I was coming. He was chanting over a small fire. When I went into the water his chanting became a lot louder, my brother didn't know what to do. The shaman told my brother to take coals from his fire and start another fire, not too far away and put some of his dried meat on it. All this time the shaman was chanting. I had planned to drown myself in the lake. His chanting seem to just pull me out of the water. After some time I came out of the lake and went and squatted then sat in front of the old shaman, he was still chanting. I don't know just how long I was there in front the old shaman. The chanting had softened into a kind of hum. He was putting something on his fire, then using a feather to push the smoke at me. It seems that my hurt was leaving me, this came to me that Running Deer would not have wanted me to do this. I believe the old man had brought her spirit to tell me this. When I came out of my daze I went over where my brother was and lay down till morning sun came up. When I came to my brother was fixing some food, he also had a water bag next to me. I was much relieved. My Indian tracker friend was also there he had followed on foot. He knew I hadn't take any weapons and he'd wanted to make sure I was safe. He was also going to go into the water and pull me out. My brother told him the old shaman told him he was taking care of it. I would be coming out of the water by myself. They had observed the whole ceremony. Being spiritual they knew and trusted the old shaman. I wanted to thank the old shaman but he had already left. My brother and tracker said they didn't see the old shaman leave.

I could tell my brother and my tracker friend were glad to see me back to something like my normal self. We headed back to the village again at a leisurely pace. My brother was very quiet he never spoke all this time nor did my tracker friend, they wanted me to come out of the shell I was in and talk first. I began by thanking him for being with me and also said this is the second time you aided in saving my life. I also thanked my tracker friend for being so loyal. We then just walked side-by-side when we could then single file with me in the middle when the trail narrowed. I felt a wonderful surge of love for these two and also the chief. Both men told me the chief wanted to come but he had been warned that some others were scouting our village. They knew we had a lot of trading supplies. He knew that if he had left with some other of his Braves, the village would have been raided. When we got to the village I went up and thanked the chief, he acted like he didn't know what I was talking about. He could have held both men back especially when he knew they might be raided. I told him I was now all right, the old shaman had help me to get rid of my hurt. Then we sat down and decided we would do about the ones that were scouting the village. The other two trackers were out looking and found the main party, there were not lot of them.

One tracker's were out and were keeping an eye on the three scouts that were watching the village. The chief decided we would wait till morning daybreak. Then move in on the main party next morning. Looked like they were getting ready to leave. To make sure they were leaving we then also showed ourselves. They then really scramble to leave in a hurry, even leaving some of their belongings behind. We were glad we didn't have to put up a fight to drive them off.

The next morning the Chief called us together for a counsel .We didn't have any dogs in the village. The garden the woman had planted were being raided by other animals, we needed dogs to keep the varmints away from the plantings. Just a few days before three Braves had stopped for a visit, this is when we found out that another village had a lot of puppies. They would probably be glad to get rid of some of them without too much trading.

Everyone was excited about going for a visit and acquiring dogs again. It had been some time since the rabies outbreak that took the chief's wife and child and two other children. The chief knew we needed the dogs to guard our plantings, but also they put up a ruckus when strangers were around. We had been fortunate that some of the younger boys were out on a make-believe raid and had discovered one of the scouts without him spotting them. We needed dogs for quite a few things. He told me they had eaten dog when food had been real scarce. Some would have starve if not for the dogs. I never knew on the farm why we didn't have a dog. Most farms had one or two, I decided would ask my mom why, when I returned to the farm.

Set out for the other village everyone enjoying the trip still didn't have enough horses so we all walked. The woman had everything we needed for food and shelter, this was brought along by the poll drags on the horses. The chief and the rest of us went out hunting for fresh meat. The third day out we were able to kill two deer. This was a welcome feast from o eating traveling food. Another two days of traveling we found the village had moved. Our main party hadn't gotten to where the other village had been. We stopped and waited for the scouts to locate their trail and where they headed. The tracker scattered out to locate their village and trailed to the new village and find the quickest way there. Within a couple of hours we were all back and had found the old village and the trail to the new. The Chief sent our trackers out to let them know we were coming to trade. . Another day of steady walking we caught up to the other village. We also had seen buffalo. A hunt was arranged and off we went to try and have at least one for our entrance into the village.

My tracker friend came to me and my brother. Neither of us had been on a buffalo hunt before. They then told us just watch and see how it was done. It could be very dangerous but if you knew what to do it was much easier and less dangerous. They walked on the opposite side of their horses keeping themselves hidden, the Buffalo had been hunted before with men on horseback and would immediately take flight. When they got in range they quickly mounted with bows on the ready. Gonacheaw was into the small herd and had got his arrow off, he then just followed until the animal dropped. His arrow had gone through the lungs. The animal running was not long before it bled out and dropped. One of the other Braves was also successful. We had two Buffalo to enter the village with. They were glad to see us. The chief had relatives here I had thought this was the village that had the dogs for trade. The village that had the dogs for trade were only a half day's ride away. We had a big feast and enjoyed the evening festivities.

The next day Our chief decided to just take some of the men to do the trading. We arrived at this village it seemed as though they were very unfriendly and subdue. I felt an uneasy feeling when entering. Most villages we came into always had a big welcome.

The chief said he would trade for six dogs, after much bickering we had two females and four male dogs. While the deal had been concluded, they sat down with our Braves for a general confab to catch up on all the other news. I wasn't much interested in taking part in. I got up and made my way to the latrine found this village not as clean as the others we had stopped at. The dogs were quite subdue I could see why they were treated very cruelly. The one we were trading with was a sub chief and when a dog got in his way he kicked it or hit it with a stick he was carrying. My feelings toward this man were not good. Getting ready to leave one of the small dogs we had traded for got loose and came to me and sat at my feet. I was still feeling grief from losing my bride, I stepped around him, and he just followed me and would then sit when I stopped. The dog actually adopted me. I still tried to look nonchalant, this is when the sub chief had been watching me. He then told our Chief That Was not one of the Dogs. My chief then told him the deal

A Past Life: as told by Brave Hawk

had been closed. Then the sub chief bristled up and said he would kill the dog before it left the village. This got my dander up and I knew I would have fought for this little dog. My chief then stated your life or the dogs. We will leave with the dogs or your life will be forfeit. All our men were on their feet and ready for what was to come. The sub chief just backed down.

We then gathered up the dogs and left. I decided to pick this dog up and carry him on my horse until were well away from this village. Some of the Braves stayed behind us and one each of our outside. Our chief said they might try to ambush us because he made them back down. We also knew the chief's reputation had preceded us. All the Braves were surprised that the sub chief had tried such a stunt. One of the outriders came in very leisurely, He informed us that some of the other Braves from the tribe had ridden hard to get ahead of us. He said there were only four, we had six. If they caught us by surprise it would even things out they figured. It was hard for me to understand how they knew this land so well. The Braves all knew this country well. Our Indian village had been moved many times over the years. The land was like my backyard to them. The chief and Braves knew where they would try. The chief then divided us up we would take them by surprise.

My brother and myself went with the head tracker. The chief and the others went off to the left, we rode leisurely about an hour or so. Our tracker stopped and we dismounted. The dogs and horses had been secured where we could come back for them. We then went on foot and kept ourselves pretty well concealed. The chief and the others had gotten there ahead of us and two of their braves were dead from arrows, the other two had escaped. Chief said the sub chief was one of the ones who had escaped. We will have to watch ourselves because he will eventually try again in the future.

The Braves retrieved their arrows and other weapons they then left the dead Braves for the buzzards. We believe someone from their village would come out to get them. We then went back to retrieve the dog and horses. The dog that had adopted me just didn't act like the others, he was like an older dog. Just came over and sat by my feet. Did not try to lick me didn't even wag his tail. The chief and the other said this dog has adopted you and your will have to adopt him.

I never had a dog before. When younger and on the farm I had asked my mom for one, my father for some reason would not have a dog around. This was a new experience for me. The village figured the dog knew I needed some type of close companion. This dog was very intelligent, couldn't get over how after going to the latrine he would do the same he never messed in the village like the other pups did. Took some time to teach them to go outside the village to do their business. They weren't exactly cruel with the dogs but were very firm. Within two weeks they had them all trained to Go outside of the village. The children were having a ball with the young dogs. Just having them around seemed to brighten the village up.

We had made a few trips back to the trading post I had helped start. We traded hides and Indian goods for hardware and other things wool blankets were well received also beads and other trinkets. Some of the Braves enjoyed the trinkets as much if not more than the woman.

This time Chum was there and we had a good long talk, he said I acted more Indian now. He could see some of my sparkle was gone. I then told him about losing my bride how devastated I was. Then how the old Shaman had called me out of the lake and relieved me of much of my pain. I had not got back to see him to thank him. One day this would happen I just knew. Chum told me mom Sue and Chuck were Asking for me would like to see me again. The two blacksmiths always ask how well I was faring.

The chief said to me, I should go back and if I decide to stay it was okay. I was part of his village and always would be, he made it plain I never would have to ask I would always be welcome. I was

A Past Life: as told by Brave Hawk

part of his tribe and a cousin by my adoption, I could never ask for a better friend and companion.

I knew that the chief and the others Braves were planning a raid on a Pawnee village that had a lot of horses. One of our best trackers and Scout was watching the village. It wasn't as far away as we had originally thought. Two days steady ride would take us there. I just couldn't miss this raid.

I decided that the next time we came in to trade I would then go back to see Chuck mom and Sue Our village not having enough horses and not able to trade for them the price was always high and never got the better ones in a trade. My best friend the tracker had scouted the village and they had 20 or more ponies. They kept a close watch on them. After watching for a few days he had found one of their weaknesses. At dawn the men guarding the ponies, would leave and go into the village to eat. This happened every day, we had a good hour to get into position and make our move. The ponies were in a rope corral which wasn't very substantial. We knew if we were to get on the back of one we could stampede the rest of them through the ropes. None were actually tied. Being one of the better riders I was chosen to make the start of the raid. Not too much to worry about, no one was watching. They had gotten over confident and had left their guard down. The other trackers and Braves were waiting and once they see us driving the ponies they would join us. We would do our best to keep them herded so they wouldn't scatter. We knew if they scattered we would lose a good share of them. I had left my filly and dog with the others. I had made the dog know he wasn't to follow me he stayed with the other Braves very reluctantly. The chief and I moved into the position. When he gave the signalled we both made our move. The ponies were used to having different men around so we didn't really disturb them that much when we entered the corral. Then we just cut the ropes and mounted the best looking pony. The chief had done the same thing. We then let out a few war-hoops to get them all going. We're they ever ready to run, we couldn't believe how well everything was going. Our Braves were ready and joined us in the run. We glance back could see the men in the village, could tell they were really upset.

As we rode I whistled for my filly she came running up alongside me with my dog following on the run. I transferred over to my filly, even though riding bareback all my life I was much more comfortable riding my own mare. She knew my every move didn't need reins.

We had lost about a third of the horses in our first mad dash away from the village. We slowed down but kept Moving all night. Next morning we kept riding but not hard, the ponies had had their run and were calmer and quite easy to control. About midday one of our outriders said he had seen some one or maybe two moving ahead of us. I then moved to the front of the ponies with the chief. Flanked the ponies on the left and right. Wasn't long before we came over small hill two Pawnee Braves came charging at us. I pulled my knife and my tomahawk, then raced toward him so he wouldn't scatter the ponies. The chief did the same with the other. As I rode toward the other brave I could see he had his tomahawk in his left hand. He was moving to my right side me being right-handed would be at a disadvantage. Just as we were getting real close made my filly moved to his left. As we came together, I raise my left hand with the tomahawk and my knife in the right hand. As we met he quickly lowered his tomahawk into a backhand swing I had also turned and stabbed and caught him in the chest. His tomahawk hit me in the lower left side breaking ribs. We both stopped, me close to passing out from the blow. He just sat on his pony than just slumped down and fell off. The chief had wounded the other brave and then driven him off. We realized there were only two Braves because it was all the ponies they could catch.

Chief came over he knew I was hurt quite bad. Blood was running down unto my hip. My shirt had protected me some. They wanted me to dismount I refuse and told him to go ahead I would follow at a walking pace, I couldn't stand any jolting. The chief left my brother and my best friend with me. They tied the brave I had killed on his pony and headed him back toward the Pawnee village. I just lost track of time but was glad to see our village.

The old shaman, the chief's father, was also a healer. I got off my pony went in to his tepee. The woman helped to get my shirt off. I was still in a lot of pain but not near as much. In order to see the extent of the damage he had hot water brought in to wash off all the caked blood. He then had me drink something and also he put something in the small fire he had going and had me inhale this. He then asked me if I was spitting blood. My answer was no. He nodded to let me know that was a good thing. He then checked out my wound found one of the ribs was underneath the other one. He then used a small stick with a hook on the end. He then slid it in and pulled the rib back into place. Whatever he gave me to drink and sniff had eased the pain. Then I was packed with some kind of Herb and then wrap tightly with the leather band. He had a kind of back frame and had my brother drive a couple of stakes in the ground inside the tepee and set the back frame up. This was so I could relax. My Indian mother and the chief's mother hovered over me like a couple of hens laying Eggs. Within a week I was back on my feet and recovering well. The old shaman was amazed at how fast my wound was healing.

Hadn't seen my own mother and Aunt Sue and Chuck for quite some time. Made up my mind I would go back if nothing else for a visit. How long I would stay I wasn't sure. We needed trading supply so we went back with the trading furs and a few buffalo hides in tow. My luck held again Chum was there at the post, he welcomed all of us set up a feed from the stores he had brought with him. He anticipated we might come in to trade he had been there a couple of weeks hoping I would show up. Mom had told him for me to come home to take care of things, she missed me and prayed I was okay. The chief made the trade for what he and the others wanted, they then wanted a lot of trinkets and beads. They also love the wool blankets. I now was wearing all buckskin, still had my linen underwear clean but they were getting quite ragged.

This is when I made up my mind to go back and see my other family, told the chief he understood. As we made our departure, my brother I could see was upset about me leaving, also my good friend Gonacheaw was also upset. I then realize how close we had become. Told them I definitely would be back. Just a nodded to acknowledge my words was all the answer they gave. By now I was very fluent in their language.

We made good time on the way back. Chum couldn't get over my dog sticking close to me all the time. The dog wasn't one that showed affection but was always by my side. We travelled at a fast pace Chum had hired men to haul the carts so we didn't have to wait for them. This cut our travel time in half or Less.

Mom Chuck and Aunt Sue were thrilled to see me. They could tell I was a lot more subdue, they wanted to know all about my goings-on. Then had to tell them about losing my bride and how the old shaman had called me out of the large lake. He had chanted over me most of the night. I told how I went into a deep sleep and had woke to find my Indian brother and very good friend Gonacheaw there. They were going to go into the lake to pull me out. The shaman told them he would call me back, if he could not then he would leave them go in and get me. I came out on my own because of his calling, he had also relieved me of much by pain. Mom and Aunt Sue said my bride would never have wanted me to do that. I said that I knew that now. Had to tell them how happy I had been, how the whole village had enjoyed me being with them. Had to tell about my adoption and my younger brother and how he had saved me from getting arrowed. How I had knocked both arrows out of the air. No one could believe I did such a thing without my spiritual protection. Also how he and my tracker friend watched over me at the lake. I told them I now had two wonderful families.

Chuck mom and Sue said I had to go into the village to see their bookkeeper. Mom said it was an all time job keeping up with everything. Mom and Chuck had hired a man from the city to do all the book work and billing of all the commodities. The sawmill was doing very well. It had expanded quite a lot since I had seen it. Mom told me to go into the village first and the bookkeeper will tell you what is going on. I had no idea of the way things had expanded. The farm was going well but was now just one of the money-makers. Chuck said he had sold the blacksmith shop two the men who were now running the blacksmith shop part ownership he knew I wouldn't mind, Chum was happy about it also. He kept the rights to do special work when we wanted to. Now we let them have the profits except for very small percentage

My dog was also my constant companion I now had grown very fond of him. He would follow or trot alongside of my filly. Mom and Sue had agreed to let him in the house he was so well behaved. He would lay at my feet or to my side or wherever I sat. Told him to stay somewhere just point and tell him to lay down. This was done in the Indian language. Mom and Sue would ask me what I had told him to do. They were amazed at how well behaved he was.

Next day went into the village which had grown quite a lot in size. Found my way okay, the bookkeeper was expecting me. Chuck had something to do with him and told him I would be in to see him. He was to give me all the information and answer all my questions. I had found I was included as a partner in all the things that Chuck and Chum had been up to. They had established a bank account in the city with two reputable banks. Chuck was shrewd and knew the best places for any of our earnings. The trade with the Indians was very profitable, also the sawmill was a going concern. Now had 4 or 5 full-time workers at the mill. One of the men was doing a lot of the repairs who is very good at this we. Needed someone like this to keep the mill running. Chum said bird you would have been perfect for the job with all your ideas.

The bookkeeper informed me I was a third partner. The holdings we had now were quite substantial. It was hard to believe that there was that much money in the accounts. There was a major account and three separate ones. The separate ones were Chuck Chum and myself. A percentage from the major account was put into each account. The major account was also used for all the expenditures that came up so our personal accounts weren't touched. I was amazed at how Chuck and mom had set everything up. We were now considered very rich. I just had to sign some papers and everything would be done I needed to do this in the city. What a wonderful feeling to have father-in-law and a brother of this caliber.

The bookkeeper had eyes on my dog who came in with me. I had to explain he was well behaved. Also I added just kiddingly, my dog only tore someone's throat out only on my command. The bookkeeper's eyes got very large and I had a hard time convincing him I was just kidding. I had him pet my dog and see that he was very friendly. For some reason he seemed to know if a person wasn't trustworthy. How he knew this I had no idea. He readily accepted the bookkeeper's pat.

When we finish decided to go to the blacksmith shop and see my old friends there. They heard I was in town and were expecting me. Had to have a glass of cider and some of their wives pastry. They wanted me to stay for the noon meal. I stayed even though I was anxious to get back to see the sawmill and other changes. After the meal they took me aside, and told me about the man that I threaten to cut his throat last time I was here. He was somewhat of a braggart and told his cronies he would take care of me. Thanked both the men and their wives and took my leave. I also made sure my dog had some food and water.

The horses were no problem having numbers of them at the shop for shoeing. My pony was still munching on some grain they had put out for her. She acknowledged me right away. Still road

A Past Life: as told by Brave Hawk

without saddle. Use a harness to hold my rifle and other things I carried, I was quite recognizable. Being only one that had ever seen with a knife on their shoulder. From the time before the word had gotten around if you had any nasty remarks they had better be where I couldn't hear them. As we were heading out of the village a few children were watching me and my dog. Out of my side vision seen to bigger boys pick up stones I knew what they plan, spun my pony around and with two jumps was standing in front of them, my dog came up and growled, they immediately drop the stone. This is when I said if you boys had thrown those stones and hit my horse or worse yet had hit my dog he would have tore your throats out. Their eyes told me how scared they were. I informed them this was an Indian dog and didn't put up with such antics. Now if you boys would like to make friends with me and him we will shake hands and you can pet my dog. They readily agreed. They then wanted to know if I was an Indian, told them no but I lived with them for some time they were very good people. There were some bad ones, there was also a lot of bad whites also. A lot more bad whites. They were a lot like us only they lived differently. Hunted for their living all the time. I wanted to make friends with the children not enemies, so I just squatted down and told them about some of my exploits. I left out any gory things told mostly about hunting. Other children had gathered also and were fascinated by my stories. I couldn't get over how much I was enjoying myself. One of the boys was quite reserved. When it was time for me to go I called my pony but before I could mount this boy tugged at my sleeve. Not knowing what was wrong or what he wanted I turned and asked them what I could do for him. This is when he told me he had heard a man bragging he was going to take care of me. He also told me he had taken his rifle and left down the road he knew I would be taking. The other boys and girls were all nodding. This surprised me this man was going to try and ambush me. Thought about taking a different route home decided to heck with it keep my eyes and ears open. Hunting and tracking with my Indian friends it taught me to watch far anything out of place or any out of place movement. They had shown me all the things that were natural and what movements that were also a giveaway. A deer flicking and ear or tail gave them away even though they were well camouflaged. When I was on the alert like this my dog also came alive very watchful. On the road there were a lot of places that he could hide. Watched carefully each place where he might hide. I knew he would be along here somewhere after being warned by the kids I just had befriended. Didn't dare relax my vigilance even though no outward sign so far. Was still being very watchful. Just ahead there was a big clump of trees I caught a movement and also heard the click of a gun be in cocked. Quickly dropped off my pony. I had prepared ahead of time that my rifle would be ready if needed. The shot came just as I had made my move to drop off my pony, my dog with my motion charge into the brush. The man was trying to reload my dog hit him, he began screaming. Racing in pointed my rifle at his head called my dog off. Then knocked him aside the head and tied his hands behind his back. Took some rope that I always carried in the loop around his neck. Picked up his rifle and turned him back toward the village. People came out when they see me coming with him and I explained he had just tried to gun me down. Surprising to me they had a holding cell, by this time it was mid-afternoon kind of spoiled the rest of my day. Another surprise was that one of the blacksmith brothers was also there village justice

They then asked me what had happened. The justice had gathered a bunch of people they had been sworn in on his Bible. They listen to me then to him he tried his best to tell him I had sicked my dog on him and showed the bites. The people knew this man from all those stunts he had pulled on them and had lied to get out of it. They asked me again how it happened. Then told them about the kids that had warned me. Another man also add he had told others he was going to get me. By this time it was late in the afternoon. The jury, the judges sworn in would be the ones who decided his fate. I was surprised they all agreed to hang him. He started to yell and cry, less than an hour went by and he was hung on a Very Large Tree in the Village. I was very glad I had not killed him back where he had ambush me. My reputation soared they

A Past Life: as told by Brave Hawk

knew I could have done him in without much questioning.

His belongings were offered to me turned all down told the justice to see that the kids all got to share of what was sold by the justice. He said to me that will make you some good friends with the parents and the kids.

Now I had to go back to the farm and tell them what happened and why I was so late in getting back to the farm. Mom and Aunt Sue were very upset to think someone in village would try to do me in. Chuck and Chum just grin and told mom and Sue if he had known my reputation he would never have tried tangling with me. I had to laugh because I didn't think I was that tough. Mom and Sue had to give me a big hug.

Made up my mind to get up to the sawmill and next day. Went out to check on my pony one of the farmhands had already fed and watered curried her down. He said she was a wonderful little filly. I told him he didn't have to take care of my horse. He smiled and said it was his pleasure he love horses and all animals. He then asked me to tell him about the Indians when I had time someone had came and told him and others what had happened in the village. I told him didn't know that they would just hang him. Again he smiled told me the villagers would have found some way to get rid of him. He had caused so much trouble by his lying about others got some in trouble and they were innocent luckily could prove it. They knew he was stealing. When he stole something he would go elsewhere to sell his ill-gotten gains. He had not been caught in the act as yet. This was the first time he got caught in a very serious crime.

Next morning Chum said he would go up with a sawmill with me he knew how I liked the building and also figured out what to do and how to do it. I was surprised that all the improvements and the expansions. Circular saw blade had been installed for sawing the smaller boards etc. The wooden shafted driven machinery had been replaced with a steel one. The carriage had metal straps on the rails made for a smoother running carriage. Didn't know any of the men, Chum introduced me to them they all started to talk at once then laugh. They then nodded to one of the men to do the talking. He then asks if some of the things they had heard about me were true. I had no idea of what they had heard. Chum stood there with a big grin on his face. I don't know what stories he had told them. Chum gave me a slight nod and then said they were true. Still not knowing what they were referring to. They then had to question me about my encounter with a man who had just been hung. Had to relate the whole story of how I had threatened to cut his throat last time was here. So he had held a grudge. Thanks to the kids telling me what they had heard him bragging about and also seen him leave the village with his rifle. I knew he was out there somewhere didn't tried to explain the lessons but Indian trackers had taught me. Probably would have been shot if not for their teachings and the kids warning. I knew every slight movement that was supposed to be nature moving them. You always look for things out of the ordinary. I caught the movement plus the cocking of his rifle. The second he raised his rifle I was off my filly and his shot missed. Then sicked my dog on him.

Leaving a sawmill headed back to the farm. Mom and Sue were in the herb garden. They came in the house with us to have the noon meal. Chuck and Chum had devised the metal fireplace, more like a stove. The top was flat to put kettles and pans on. There was always hot water on the stove. Later looking at it I suggested putting doors on. Chum laughed and said bird Chuck and I were in the process of doing just that at the smith shop. He said this time were one step ahead of you.

Was greatly amazed at how much the village had expanded. Chuck and Chum had to run people off our land. They then put up post every so often to let people know they were trespassing. We didn't mind them walking or berry picking, but made sure they will refrain from trying to build on our land.

Mom Chuck Chum and aunt Sue, told me after the evening

A Past Life: as told by Brave Hawk

meal we want to discuss our holdings and what they have been doing with the money that had been earned from the farm the sawmill in the trading post we had done well the profits from just the Indian trading for hides skins had brought good returns. They then told me I must go into the city and establish myself at the banks. They would need my signatures and would want to establish who I was visibly.

I agreed to go into the city. Chuck said he would accompany me, he had trading and transactions to take care of. I would be welcome to accompany him two any these doings. I made no comment at the time. Knew I wasn't interested in this type of thing. When with the Indians my chief and some of the others including my best friend tracker and brother would do all the dickering.

My dog was my concern now, I didn't want to take him into the city. I knew he would follow me where I went. Mom and Sue said they would keep him for me. We decided to put him in a pen until I had been gone for a couple of days. Felt bad for my dog he had never been penned was always free to come and go as he pleased. I could tell he liked mom Chum Chuck and Chum. He would go to mom and Sue for a pet then back to his place I had made for him. He would just lay on one of my old buckskin shirts. Mom and Sue couldn't get over how he would follow my every move, if I headed outside he was at my side. Took my shirt out and put it in the pen. He seemed to know that he was to lay in there, he went over and lay down. He looked at me as if to say what did I do to deserve this. I normally didn't show him an awful lot of affection. Couldn't help myself squatting down and rubbing his ears and petting him.

Had everything ready for my trip. Chuck was checking on our horses. The men working in the barn had a brought them out. Chuck's horse was saddled, the men wanted to know where my saddle was, laughing told them never used a saddle road bareback since I was a kid. How in heck do you stay on one of the young men asked me. Just comes natural if you've done it all the time.

I picked up my traveling things, this was what I carried in front of me. Also had a pack on my filly's rump for traveling. Chuck said I would be surprised at how the trail had been improved over the years. There were now taverns along the way. He never used them, they were filthy with vermin and weren't very clean. Our pack horses carry our sleeping and lean to in case of rain. Everything went well we were in the city a lot sooner than I thought we would be.

Chuck was going to come to the bank with me. Told him just to tell me where to go and you can take care of your business. He laughed, then told me about caring my knife would kind of rattle the bankers. Also if I wore it I may be challenge. There were some very unsavory men seem to delight in a knife fight. Usually someone was found dead after an encounter. Told Chuck I would feel naked without my knife.

Stabled our horses, Chuck assured me they were very good with horses. He tipped them well so they were always exceptionally caring with our horses Chuck left in their care.

We went to the inn and left our sleeping and other baggage. Chuck headed into the trading places he needed to go. Heading me toward the bank. I found I was getting a lot of staring because of my attire. I guess I look something like an Indian. The bank was a masonry building and it looked very substantial.

Walked into the entrance and about 10 steps in and stopped for a look around. Everyone had turned and actually stared. This tickled the heck out of me. I had a hard time keeping a straight face. Finally a clerk came out from somewhere in the back and asked me if I was in the right place informing me this was a bank. He said I should leave I just gave him a hard look trying to hold back a big grin. Then informed him I would not have entered if I had been in the wrong place. This kind of shook him up and he stuttered, shifting from 1 foot to the other. Decided to put him out of his misery. Told him who I was here to see. He his eyes kind of bugged out, he took off and went into the back. Next came out

A Past Life: as told by Brave Hawk

an elderly man with a big grin on his face. Then he motioned me to follow him into his office. He had been expecting me because Chuck had told them I would be in some time when I got back from my trading forays.

He then said he was just outside of the office when I walked into the bank, he had not seen the patrons or his teller so rattled in a long time. He then said I knew right off who you were. Just wanted to let things play out, not too much excitement in the bank. This will be talked about for quite a while. He told me Chuck had told him about some of my exploits and he would welcome me to his home if only I would come. He introduced himself as John and we shook hands.

Now he said I have everything ready for your signature. He then said he didn't want to insult me but asked if I could read and write. Informed him my mom dad and aunt had taught me well. He then had someone get the paperwork. Then went through explaining what was going on. This was part of all the business Chuck and he had established. There was a tidy sum involved. Then told him had to go to the other bank shrugging my shoulders to let him know I wasn't much interested in the financial affairs. Told him I had made a promise to mom Chuck and Aunt Sue and I would do what they asked. He then asked if he could accompany me. I readily agreed. He said when we get there that he would not go in with me at first. Wanted to see if I shook up the other patrons and tellers like I had in his bank. We were able to walk to the other bank, wasn't just a short distance away. Opened the door and stepped in and took about 10 steps and stopped to look around. Again everyone stared. Then one of the tellers came out to meet me in a gruff voice told me I was in the wrong place and had best leave. Just gave him a hard stare and then he got very agitated and proceeded to call for one of the guards. This is when my banker who came over with me walked in and took my arm and escorted me into the other banker's office. He was chuckling all the way in. The other banker stood up and welcomed us, asking what the commotion was out in the bank my banker John told him one of his tellers wanted to throw me out until he intervened. They both had a big chuckle over this. We shook hands and he introduced himself as Orrin He said he knew who he was and would reprimand him. I said no absolutely not please invite him in I would like to meet him formally. He was just doing his job as he could see it. The banker sent for him and he came in I believe he thought he would be fired or demoted. When he came in I stood up and offered by hand, he was surprised and was very pleased to shake hands. I wanted to make friends not enemies. Then asked him to sit down with us this was not normal thing that was done. He had been afraid of me and had thought he was taking the right actions. He was told by the banker who I was. He said he knew our charts well and had wondered who the other patron was. He got up and went out to bring in the paperwork also the papers I needed to sign. He grinned and said that I had shook up his patrons and tellers. He was ahead teller, I had taught him a lesson don't Judge by an appearance.

Asked him what he did with his leisurely time, he said he got out of the city is much as possible.

Did a little hunting lived alone wife passing a few years previously. I just seem to know that we had something in common. I invited him to our farm when he had any time he could spare. He was very gracious and said if he could he would accept my invitation I had also extended an invitation to the two bankers.

When our business was completed they invited me out to an exclusive eating place that only the elite were allowed to enter. I didn't know this at the time it was more of a show and tell situation my attire and appearance were to spark some excitement for the bankers and other patrons. They said they would have something to talk about for some time. Off we went as we started to enter they had me go first they knew that the guard would confront me. Sure enough a large man stepped out to stop me. He looked me up and down then just told me to go in. The two bankers then showed up,

A Past Life: as told by Brave Hawk

they couldn't figure out why the guard had let me in. I knew what was going on I signalled to the guard with my eyes letting him know someone was behind me. He thought it was some kind of a prank the two bankers were playing on him and the others. Dressed in buckskin and wearing a knife on my shoulder and Tomahawk on my hip was something they had never seen. My appearance was not shabby, did not wear a hat my hair was tied back neatly in a ponytail. I use the herbs my bride had taught me to use so I didn't give off an offensive odor. The head waiter came and asked who I was with, the banker showed themselves and we were escorted to their private table. They ordered I just shrugged my shoulders. The head waiter said he would bring something special for me and I agreed. Two bankers were getting a charge out of all the glances we were receiving they told me this was one of the better days for them. He gave them something other than banking they could talk about with other diners at a later date. The meal was excellent I complemented the waiter and also the cook

Both bankers knew I had been out with Indians for some time. I told them yes I was now able to speak and understand their language. Questioning me did I not have any Indian friends. Had to tell them the chief was a very good friend also had a Indian brother who had save my life and had watched over me and also my tracker friends. Most white men at the time were not accepted I was an exception. Told them my story how I was caught and I escaped and how I was accepted didn't tell about the spiritual part that I had told the Indians. Took all afternoon almost evening. Then I said I had to leave. They were fascinated with my stories didn't want me to leave. I had had enough and said I had to leave. They asked where I was staying for me this was a very rough part of the city. They asked if I would like a couple of escorts. They could tell this upset me so didn't say any more.

Chuck would probably be having dinner before long headed off on foot to go back to my sleeping accommodations. Didn't like the city because it smelled so terrible. Was later than I had thought it was already getting dark. Halfway to the inn I could sense some one or two were following me. Even in the city my senses were acute. Turned the corner stopped pulled my knife and Tomahawk out on the ready. Could hear running down another alley, they were running ahead to cut me off and surprised me. I then stayed out in the middle the alley. Actually sensed where they were, there footsteps and breathing hard gave them away. As I got to the other crossing alley one came at me with a knife in his hand and thought to stab me in the gut. Was already prepared Tomahawk caught his knife hand my knife buried in his chest, the other man tried to hit me with his club, made a quick dodge and spun and slashed his throat and backed away. They would never attack anyone again. Then headed back to the inn. Chuck was waiting supper for me, told him of my days with the bankers. Then told him I just killed two men shook his head check me over and asked if I was hurt. I was used to this type of a fight. I had sparred with my Indian tracker who taught me a lot also I thanked Chuck for his original teachings

We ate then Chuck said we would go to the police of the city, to let them know what had happened. He said this way word would get out you wouldn't be anyone to trifle with. So off we went the young officer was fairly new. He asked if I was confessing to killing these two men. I raise my eyebrows and said of course I killed them before they could kill me. Chuck stepped in and told him he had better get his boss and now before we threw him out on his ass. He decided he had better get his boss. The officer that came in looked recognized Chuck and gave him a smile and ask what the problem was. Then we related what happened well was his answer, you're lucky to be alive. We know who they are they and said were quite sure they were behind quite a few murders. Had not had any real proof as yet now they didn't need any. He then told the young officer get some help and go pick up the bodies. I didn't care much for this young officer he acted like he was on the shifty side.

The two bankers John and Orrin had invited me and Chuck to

A Past Life: as told by Brave Hawk

supper at their houses. We decided we weren't that much of a hurry to get back to the farm so we accepted the invite. Chuck told me be careful he heard that a rumor was out that one of the toughs was looking to catch me and challenge me to a knife fight. I was always with my knife and carried the Tomahawk also. Where ever I went they were with me. Went to check on my filly to see how she was doing. In town my dog was with her. the hostler told me he found the dog with my filly. He must be mine. He told me he had fed and watered him and he curled up and stayed with my filly.

I was amazed that my dog could have traced me into the city. He was glad to see me came to me and just sat next to my leg. I stooped down and gave him a good petting. Normally would have just patted him on the head. The hostler was standing watching, I spoke Indian to the dog and made them stay with my filly. Then asked the young hostler to feed my dog and he readily agreed. He also asked me what kind of language I was speaking. I told him that was Indian that I had learned when I lived with the Indians. Then told him my dog only understood Indian he would stay with my filly, he had been taught on hunting and scouting forays he was meant to stay with the horses. He understood when I told him to stay with my filly.

I decided to just wander around the city for something to do and to explore some of the goings-on in the city. Was interested in a big blacksmith shop and wanted to see if they had anything new to learn. Walked in and met one of the workers. He asked if he could do something for me. Told him I did some black-smithing a while back and wonder if there was anything new going on. They had used the waterwheel also now thinking of a steam engine. Had devised quite a lot more tools that were powered. They were able to make sheeting using rollers that were designed to be adjustable. This was quite interesting for me. This was used to make the pots and frying pans cups etc. Chuck did a lot of our buying from this shop.

By the time I got back to the inn, Chuck was waiting for me and off we went to John the bankers houses. He had to be doing well for his home was exceptionally well done. The wood work was beautiful. They offered drinks of any kind. I enjoyed the sherry, I had one drink and when I finish they wanted to give me a refill. Turned it down, the one drink satisfied me. I didn't like the feeling or the effects of alcohol and refrained from drinking. We spent the evening talking in general some about banking and others of our farm and experience with the saw mill and trading.

The bankers turned to me and said now we would like to hear about some of your experiences. Chuck laughed and said you won't believe how he was captured and escaped. Then was accepted and adopted into the tribe. I began my story and when I was done with that they wanted me to tell more. I said will do so next time. It was time for us to leave for the evening it was quite late by this time. Chuck also wasn't a drinker either he would have one or two drinks then that was all for him. We headed back to the inn and had a good night's rest. Chuck asked if I would like to accompany him on his next trading foray, to me it was boring so I declined.

Chuck was off on his trading forays. I just decided to wander around and check on my filly and dog. The Hostler said he took my filly out for a short ride morning and afternoon. He said my dog would follow them and would stay with the filly in the stable. He also said my dog wouldn't make up to anyone. When I walked in he knew I was there right off would get up to greet me. The Hostler said he knew I was coming because the dog was alert he must know my walk. He couldn't get over how well behaved he was. I gave him a good tip, that he did not want to take but I insisted. He was going out of his way to accommodate me. I could also see that he loved animals. I mentioned this, he smiled and said they are a lot more trustworthy and people, I had to agree.

When I left I knew someone was following me. Got this sense feeling, I believe they had come from my tracker friends he always

A Past Life: as told by Brave Hawk

knew when someone was following us also if they were friendly or not. He would ask me if I could sense this. Wasn't long I was also able to do it.

On one of our forays he told me some of the younger boys were tracking us. He then said let's see if we can fool them. We then took off our moccasins and went barefoot. He had also taught me how to hide my tracks quite well. Never step down on any foliage or grasses find somewhere to step without leaving a sign. Once learned you could move at a good pace only occasionally leaving sign we been separated and would make a loop onto our own back trail and catch them by surprise. We found them milling around where are tracks seem to disappear what a laugh we had when we walked up to them from behind. They all wanted to know how we had hidden our trail which for some time had been quite visible to them. All my tracker told them you had to walk on air I just love his sense of humor. When I was done relating this story to my Hostler friend I decided to go to the blacksmith shop. More than one was following me. The only one I know that had a grudge was the young policeman that Chuck and I had threatened to throw out on his rear. Entered the blacksmith shop and was greeted and again was shown around and things explained to me. I had a few questions and they would give me the answer as best they could they were very knowledgeable and were working with different ways of combining metals. They were very interested in my knife and my Tomahawk the Tomahawk was the one given me by the chief in my challenging fight. It was some kind of stone but well-shaped. I told them I had made the knife quite a while back. They looked it over and said it was serviceable I knew it wasn't fancy piece of work but it served the purpose it was meant to do.

When it was time for me to leave, they came out with me. Not too far off there where three men standing there. One had pulled a large knife out of his sheath and was tossing it from one hand to the other. The blacksmith wanted me to come back inside. I just shrugged and walked the few paces to meet him, already had my Tomahawk in my left hand. I knew he was right-handed when he drew his knife it was with his right hand, he went into a crouching stance. I just stood facing him, he made a few quick steps and held his knife down as he plan to gut me with it. I pulled my knife swinging my Tomahawk down knocking his hand aside and stabbing him in the arm. His knife fell to the ground, surprise was a reactionary I could see. Then laid my knife up to his throat telling him, I just gave you your life, go get your arm fixed. Next time don't let anyone crowd you into something. This is when the police officer showed up, he had a pistol in his hand. There were too many witnesses so he didn't dare to shoot. All four blacksmith came out and stood by me. He just turned around and left. Then looked at me and said he would have shot you if we had not been here. I then told them what had happened at the police station. They all laughed and said good for you. This man is no good was next comment. By the time I was done my wandering it was time for supper.

Went back to the inn and to the restaurant. Decided to sit and wait for Chuck. Wasn't long before he showed commenced to tell him my experience and knife fight. He then asked me to describe who I had fought. He nodded and said you just disarmed the best knife fighter in the area. The policeman was another matter. My comment was let's eat and worry about it when it happens Chuck said his business had been taking care of, we could leave any time I was ready.

We had one more invite to take care of. The other banker Orrin had insisted we come to his house for supper the next evening. Chuck said we didn't have to really go, I said it should be fun. Next day we took our horses out for a long leisurely ride into the countryside, what a pleasure to get away from the city for a while. Stopped at little inn. That Chuck knew and had our midday meal. My appearance always attracted attention. I accommodated any questions they might have. Had quite a gathering when I related some of my stories. Spent a pleasurable afternoon.

Heading back to the city, as we got to our inn, the police chief

A Past Life: as told by Brave Hawk

was there. He was all apologies. They had found the young police officer in the river with his head smashed in. He wanted to know if we knew anything about. We had substantial evidence of our alibis for our whereabouts. He said he wasn't worried about us, his father was well-to-do and had got him this job and was also paying his salary. His son had mentioned me and how he despised me. The old man insisted that he come and arrest me. The officer was very good friend of Chuck's. He said he would inform the old man that I wasn't anywhere around the place where they had found his son. Also my whereabouts were many miles away and was spent with friends and my partner Chuck. Chuck also said to the officer looks like he got what he was looking for. The officer just grinned, Chuck knew from encountering the man that he wasn't a very trustworthy person. Our first encounter had been threatening to throw him out of the police station on his ass.

That evening was spent at the other bankers home, he had invited quite a gathering. Found they all wanted to hear about my life with the Indians. The old man whose son had been found with his head smashed in was also there. After a while he approached me and accused me of doing his son in. I gave him a smart answer by asking was his throat cut or was he stabbed through the heart. That wasn't the case so it wasn't myself. This set the old man in a rage. This is when the bankers came and told him he had to leave. The banker's servants escorted to the door and not to gently. They then came and apologized to me. They said he was always looking for trouble when actually none existed. Didn't let this upset me, his son was the one you had to watch out for. Someone had taken care of that for all concerned. After that episode was settled the get-together went quite well. All enjoyed my stories. A few came and asked me if they were true or were they made up I just laughed and told them they would have to ask my Indian friends. Some were curious if I wore the knife and Tomahawk all the time. My answer was whenever I'm not sleeping, that got a chuckle out of most of the gathering. I also told them should have brought my dog he only knows Indian language they then had me speak Indian and asked a lot of questions. I told them they didn't have words for a lot of our things. Most had never encountered any of our things. I had told them about the sawmill, they all thought I was making up a good story for them. Then I also added you folks don't believe a lot of my stories either. That got another round of laughter. The evening ended with a lot of handshaking and welcoming to their homes.

Chuck got a big charge out of the evening. He then told me a lot of them asked him if my stories were true. He acknowledged they were all true. Some I had related they probably would not believe either. We left headed back to the inn happy the way the evening had went. I told Chuck before we leave I would like to go to the blacksmith shop. Wanted to thank them for coming down to my rescue when they saw the young police officer show up with his pistol in his hand. He didn't dare shoot me with them there. They realize what he was trying to pull off.

Next morning there was a courier with two packages. He told me they were not to be open until I got back home. I agreed to this, couldn't imagine what could be in the two packages. Chuck was also curious. He asked me if I was going to open them, I told Chuck that I had given my word I would not open them until I got home.

That morning we saddled up and went to the blacksmith shop before setting out. We had a big welcome, this is when I thanked them for being there when the police officer had shown up. They said they knew him he could see what he was trying to pull off. He didn't dare with at least four witnesses. I said we got word that they had found him with his head smashed in. Was found in some canal or other. They all agreed it was a good ending for a despicable character. My dog was with us so introduce him to them also. I couldn't get over how nonchalant my dog was, took everything in stride. After introductions he would just come back and sit by me I spoke to him in Indian, they got a big charge out of that. I said that's all he knows.

A Past Life: as told by Brave Hawk

We headed back to the farm three days riding my dog didn't have any trouble keeping up. He was used to trotting along where ever I travelled with the Indians. When we got to the farm mom and Sue were there to greet us. Seeing the dog with us were much relieved. Mom said he moped around for just a day after they fed him he disappeared, hard to believe he had found me in the city. We were in time for the evening meal. After we ate Chuck said well are you going to open those packages. The first one I opened was a smaller package, I was quite surprised so wasn't Chuck. It was the police officers pistol. We could see now why they didn't want me to open the packages and wait till we were home. Someone else would have taken it that we or I had done the officer in, because I had the pistol. Enough of a surprise now what was in the other packet. It was a knife like the one I carried on my left shoulder. This knife was one beautiful piece of work. The note said I was to start wearing it not for hanging on the wall. Even the sheath was beautifully made. Why the blacksmith had done this for me I just didn't know. Would go out of my way if and when I went back to the city to thank them.

Chum wasn't back from his getting things across River to the other side to get ready for another trading forays. We thought he would be back before this time. Was getting ready to go hunt him up, when he showed up. Could see he was distressed, we had been robbed on the trail to our trading post. One of the men was injured he tried to stop them and was injured in the process. This was the first time we had this happen. We had lost one cart the other one was okay. It wasn't a big bunch just two or three or they would have taken the whole load. We had two men at the trading post. They would have to be warned. I then was determined to track the culprits down. There was no way they could hide their tracks. They had probably unloaded the cart and pack on horses. Meant to leave the next morning. Made sure my rifle was clean and ready I also took the pistol my bow and a number of arrows. Had gotten to be a good shot with a bow used it whenever I could because I liked the idea of no noise.

The culprits had held our men at rifle point and had knocked one of the men in the head with the club. Then told the other they wouldn't hesitate to shoot if they interfered. Next morning Chum was going to come with me, the injured man told Chum he was going he owed them a little bump or two. I told Chum let me track them they can't hide their trail and when I find them I will come back for help. The men at the trading post need to be warned also. The injured man still had a wrap on his head I asked if he was sure he was all right. He insisted on going with me couldn't dissuade him. Packed our horses no pack horse is this time. We needed to travel light as possible. I was used to traveling light anyway. The man that came with me I hope would be a good companion. Never knew about a stranger, had met him before at the post. He had been working for Chum for quite some time. Chum said he was his best man. Was reluctant at first, but with Chum's approval I knew he was trustworthy. Next morning before dawn we were on our way. Chum was getting another lode ready and would not be too far behind with the other men. Two days out we came to where the altercation took place. The cart was left about a mile ahead, just as I had thought they had pack animals and had loaded them but stayed on the trail quite a ways. They then took to the woods their tracks were easy to follow. They apparently figured someone would follow them. We could see where they had made a camp and then split up. The man that was with me said do we split also, I said no. they are trying to throw us off. I then checked all the tracks the main ones were leaving a lot of tracks. Looking closer could tell they were loaded very light. The other trail that they were trying to hide I found they had loaded two horses but were very heavily loaded. We would follow that track. The other I knew was set up for ambush was sure of that. Man that was with me couldn't figure out how I did this. He said they all look the same to him. Wasn't about to try explaining just then. The next campfire we felt was still warm but out. We were getting close. At a good idea of where they were heading. An Indian village the chief and I had traded there before. We then left the trail and went ahead and parallel to get out in front of them the man I was with just followed me without

A Past Life: as told by Brave Hawk

question. He made a very good companion. Rode quite hard most of the morning, then cut back to find the trail. No one had passed. We would set up our ambush here. My companion asked was I sure this is the right trail I just nodded. My dog was with us, when we had ridden hard for a ways we had left him behind he caught up shortly.

The trail was the main one for other Indian villages. Had my man moved down the trail from me and keep his rifle ready and stay out of sight. They might try to fight us off. The man I was with name was Judd. I said Judd don't hesitate if they go for the rifle shoot and don't wait. Also told him to let them go by and I would confront them. Then he could make his move if Need be. Didn't have to wait much over an hour could hear them coming, I knew there were only two men. As he approached me I moved my filly onto the trail and told him to stop. The man I faced went for his rifle using my bow sunk an arrow into his chest. The man behind had also raised rifle before he could shoot Judd had shot and knocked him off his horse. Most of our goods were on their horses. This was my way of knowing they were heavily loaded. The tracks told me this, thanks to my Indian tracker friends. Now we would have only one man to contend with. Judd couldn't figure out how I knew of this. No way was I going to try to explain. The other man was a leader . He most likely had set up an ambush on the other trail. I figured he must have heard the one shot. Told Judd to take all the horses back and I would follow behind.

The other man would come back down the trail after he found where they were supposed to meet. The one shot may have thrown him off and would he would come down the trail to investigate. Was another 2 to 3 hours before he came walking in front of his horse looking for sign. I made the mistake of leaving the dead men on the trail. He spotted them and ducked off the trail. Now I was going to be a cat and mouse game. My advantage was my dog, still using my bow got off my filly and moved away from her. Gave her a light tap on the rump she moved off for a ways. My dog's ears were up telling me which direction he was coming. He had to be a good woodsman to do what he was doing my filly moving off had alerted him to her position. Waited for him to make his next move. Was sure he had grabbed his rifle. He was moving very slow and cautiously. I was well hidden with my dog by my side. His ears were up and watching. This man had made a looping circle around were my filly had made the noise. My dog kept me alert to the man's whereabouts. Waited to see if he would show himself when he saw my horse. When he stood up he was about 50 feet from my horse. He must have thought just a loose horse. I had my bow ready but he was also ready with his rifle. This is when I sicked my dog on him, he was surprised to all the sudden have a dog come afterhim. He turned to shoot my dog and I put an arrow into his throat and a second arrow into his chest. He never got a shot off. When over and picked up his rifle and it was a very fancy one. I now recognized him he was one of the men Chum had hired because he had also lived with the Indians. My dog even though he was done chewed on him for a while. I had sicked him on so let him chew a little before calling him off.

Went back to the trail and gathered up the other ponies with the rest of the trade goods. They were lightly loaded compared to the others we had stopped that morning. Started back on a quick trot my filly was ready for a little run. Had to hold her back show the other ponies could keep up. Caught up with Judd shortly, stopped set up for a meal unloaded the ponies and hobbled the ones that were strange to us. Let them feed and water by the stream Judd had stopped at. I didn't say much but Judd asked what had happened. Gave him a brief description of what happened. His next comment was he sure was glad he wasn't the one I was after. I couldn't help but laugh, then told him I had some wonderful teachers.

Told Judd would go back and stay with them for a while. Told him how good the trackers were that had taught me. I was only half as good as they were. Not only could they track had a sense of what they were tracking what they were doing and where they were going. We supped on the dry food we had brought with us. Judd I found to be a good companion he was not afraid to do his part and more of the chores. He was kind of down about killing the man back up the trail. Judd I answered he would have killed me and you without any hesitation. If you had hesitated to shoot he may have killed me or you. Living out here can be very hard at times. If I had went out just to kill a person just for the sake of killing that is entirely different. You were very fortunate they had not killed you or the other men with you when they robbed us. He then said we didn't even buried them. My comment was the buzzerds will get there fill saving us a lot of digging. Then added if we had taken time to bury the first two the other man would have caught us and we would be the ones needing to be buried. He said, I'm damn glad you're my friend and not my enemy. You think way ahead and by doing so things turn out okay.

I had to ask Judd if he had ever had to do a man in before. No but had been in quite a few fights not losing too many being a big man he used his size to fight. I then stated size doesn't make any difference to a rifle or a bow, they down large or small. He just laughed and agreed, saying he could see that after today. That evening decided to cut across and deliver the goods to our trading post instead of going all way back to the fork in the main trail.

Next morning told him of my decision and he agreed. But where was the other trail. Told him would make one with a grin. He said knowing you now were not going to get lost. After another day and night through the woods we hit the main trail about dark. We set up camp again by a stream. Took care of our horses, then ate. Less than a day were at the trading post.

Chum was already there, he said if I hadn't showed up by the days end he was going to get his men out and go looking for me and Judd. The men couldn't understand why Chum called me bird, all he said that's his name. Chum wanted to know if they had just surrendered the goods. My answer was we got them back. Judd then chimed in and said there's three dead men on the other trail. We gave them a chance to surrender but they had chosen to fight. Judd then related how I had set everything up. How we had raced ahead off the trail and came out ahead of the two men who had most of the goods. He also added how I knew it was the right trail when they had split up. He still couldn't figure it out, he would have taken the other trail which showed more horses had gone that way. Chum just smiled and shook his head knowing a good woodsman would read the sign maybe. I knew he would want to know the details in private. Judd said to the other men he was damn glad I was his friend and not an enemy. I then stated never killed a man only in self-defense. I wasn't particularly to being killed myself. This got a big laugh out of the crew

Went back with Chum we let the hired man bring the carts back to the farm .Chuck had asked how everything went did we get our goods back. Chum related Judd's story, Chuck nodded knowingly. After the episodes in the city knew I could take care of myself.

Still fascinated with the sawmill spent a lot of time at the mill. Had a few ideas to improve some of the machinery. The belts we had were much improved over the first one we had used. Everything was going smoothly had a lot of business. We were the only sawmill in the area. Also had some good men working for us.

Chum and I took time to do a little fishing we headed for our favorite Lake where the trout were plentiful. We were both much surprised it still was pristine no one had found it .Was hard to get to but worth all the trouble. Fished and built a fire and cooked fish with all other goodies we had brought. Told him how glad I was he and Aunt Sue had gotten together and how happy they were. Also Chuck and mom. Chum chimed in and said hey I'm your uncle now. He got a big laugh out of that.

Everything was going real well, Farm and sawmill and our trading Chuck said he had to go back into the city would everyone

A Past Life: As told by Brave Hawk

like to go. Mom was reluctant but Aunt Sue talked her into going. She wanted to get some more cotton and linen cloth and find some finer wool material. We had always went by horseback mom said what if we buy a lot of material. Chuck laughed and said Mary the carts and wagons are coming and going so we can always leave the bulk to be hauled back by them. There were inns along the way, we would not use any, they were all infested with all kinds of vermin. We brought our own lean to bedding etc. We use pack horses for that purpose. Everything went well. Mom of course had to leave instructions to everyone. They all do their jobs and just smiled nodding their heads. Mom was no slave driver just like things neat and clean.

The trip to the city went well had one night of rain but cleared and was pleasant. When we arrived Chuck made his rounds. When the bankers and friends heard we were in the city the invites came in fast and furious. I still dressed in buckskin with my new knife on my shoulder and my tomahawk on my left hip. I felt naked without my knife. We weren't hardly settled down at the inn when John one of the bankers showed up. He came just to make sure his was the first invite to dinner the very next evening he asked me if I had any more details to talk about. Told him not really. Sue chimed in yes he sure has. We were robbed and he got all our goods back. Telling the story meant telling the deaths of some more men. Mom and Sue had not heard about that either. Chuck had not heard the details either. I was reluctant to talk about it Judd had spread the word and Chuck had got it second hand.

Chuck hadn't pressured me into talking about the escapade. Word had gotten out that we had been robbed, and I had recovered our goods. There would be mixed company at the dinner. Had to ask if it was all right tell the story. Chuck and Chum said this is the city bird, the woman are not kept in the dark. They insisted on being in on the dinners not just the men, they enjoyed the stories and would get them first-hand not by someone else.

The next evening John the banker sent his carriage over for the woman and said we were welcomed to ride also if we didn't feel like riding our horses. Chuck Chum and I decided to walk being a pleasant evening. Told Chuck and Chum, would first thing in the morning go see the blacksmith to thank them for their gifts. We knew there would be a lot of whiskey wine in any kind of the liquor you would care to consume. Mom and Sue arrived and were escorted into the house or mansion as I saw it. We arrive shortly after and were also welcomed with enthusiasm. There was quite a gathering, mom and Sue were the center of attention. The city woman wanted to hear all about living out in the woods as they seem to envisioned the hard ship of living on the farm.

Just wandered around with a sherry drink in my hand. Everyone seemed to have a drink in hand, mom and Sue were not much at drinking they were doing the same as I Sherry in hand to keep from constantly encouraged to have a drink. Not any of the men approached me. I knew I didn't smell that bad. Asking Chuck what was I doing that they were kind of avoiding me. He laughed and said your reputation from the last time you were here in the city was much exaggerated. They heard that I had done six or eight man in also the police officer. My comment was the Indians did the same thing they also like a good story. Chuck told me to be a little more outgoing, go and introduce yourself and strike up a conversation. They were waiting for me they didn't want to approach and then be rebuffed. I could now understand being in their place I probably would feel the same.

A group of men in my age bracket were gathered in one section. Went over and introduce myself, they all offered their hand. Asked if they minded me joining them, they all told me I was more than welcome. Even though my dress was buckskin and knew it made me stand out. The cotton and linen and find wool were all on show. The woman were dressed exquisitely. Myself never seeing woman in such attire found myself staring and had to catch myself not to do this. Didn't realize the younger woman were also staring at me.

A Past Life: as told by Brave Hawk

My dress and the rumors set me out of the crowd. Hope that the old man that had a confronted me about his officer's son wouldn't show up. The banker John came over and struck up a conversation with us. Couldn't help but ask if the officers father had gotten over his tirade from the last dinner the banker then said he got over it okay on the way home in his carriage he had died. The banker said with a grin his meanest caught up with him.

Time for us to sit down to dinner. Had no idea of where we were to sit, Chuck and mom Chum and Sue went in and were escorted to the head of the table. Started to follow when two young girls one on each side took my arm and guided me to sit between them. Everyone could see how flustered I was and broke out into a good-matured laughter. Not being around any girls for so long didn't really know how to act. Made up my mind to just relax and enjoy so I did just that. They both talk to me about how my trip was to the city if anything exciting happen. Told them we had a very pleasant trip no excitement then one of the boulder girls asked me where my girlfriend or my wife was. This gave me a shot of spiritual pain for just a second. The other girl told the other that was a hell of a question to ask. She had seen my hurt which lasted only a second. My answer was my wife had died after only a year and a half of marriage. Then also added not too many beautiful girls out in the woods. They got a big kick out of my answer, it was the best time of my life, we had a lot of love for each other.

Made up my mind to relax, things went a lot smoother. Our meal again was excellent. The girls wanted me to meet their friends after the meal. We excuse ourselves and then they introduced me to quite a few of the girls. Somewhere of the giggly sort but were pleasant. One of the girls was very pushy, rebuffed her a number of times. The other girls just shook their heads. When the other girl was distracted one of the other girls that I liked rescued me, with a nod I followed her. I moved quickly to get out of the giggling gaggle of girls. She then guided me to the men's lounge, she then left me with a grin. I was determined to find out who she was. She wasn't beautiful like some of the others but was very pretty. I asked Chuck if he knew who she was. Chuck then told me her father is here, I'll introduce you. We found him talking with a couple other men.

We waited for them to notice us. They turned and welcomed us into their conversation. They asked me about my time with the Indians, just acknowledge and said I lived with them for a number of years. Chuck then said that I would like to talk with this young girl's father. We stepped aside and he had a curious look on his face. My reputation had proceeded me with a lot of exaggeration. I kind of stumbled around in my speech and finally blurted out if he would let me court his daughter. His eyes opened with surprise, he then chuckled and said, I have never had a man ask me that question. His answer was if she was willing he would give his blessing. Then he asked of all the rumors about me were true. This is my turn to grin. Told him that a lot of things get exaggerated. So what was being said I hadn't heard but told him don't believe only a small amount of what you have heard. Then asked if he would formally introduce me to his daughter. He readily agreed still with a grin.

When it came time for the evening set down, dessert and treats. I was supposed to sit with the other girls. Before we entered the dining area the girls' father stopped her and motioned her to come over. He introduced us then with a big grin told his daughter, I had asked him if I Could Court, Her. He said it was up to you daughter. It was the first-time I had seen her uncomfortable. Then she just grinned and said she would rescue me again, and come and sit with her and her two friends. Knew now that I was accepted by both father and daughter. She said that one of the other girls I had been sitting next to was set on catching me. She was very beautiful but not very sensible to my kind of reckoning. Enjoyed the evening declined to tell any story about my Indian experience. I figure they knew I had lived with the Indians for a few years. Had already at different dinners told about some of my experiences. I could see the pout on the other girls face because I hadn't sat with her and her friends. Her silly chatter had just turned me off.

Next day was spent with my filly and dog. Curried my filly and took time to check and brush my dog. Was glad he would stay with my filly when he was told to, the young hostler was amazed at how the dog obeyed. He told me the dog always knew my footsteps, the hostler said my dog brightened up and was out to greet me long before I showed up. Had noon lunch with the hostler's. Invited them to one of their eating places close by and insisted on paying for the meal the hostler that was caring for my filly and dog stayed behind they need someone to look after the customers even during lunch time. Told him would make it up to him. After heading back to the inn we were staying at, found a carriage with a driver standing by. He looked as though he had been there for quite a while. As I entered my room the girl that I had not sat with the evening before was in my room laying on my bed. I then asked her what she wanted. She jumped up putting her arms around my neck. Pride her loose and she said she was there to make me hers. Being upset just took her by the arm quite forcefully and headed her out of my door and down to the lobby. When we got to the lobby she started to put up a fuss, I took her over my knee and paddled her rear. Then took her out and put her in her carriage instructing the driver to take her home. Later that evening eating supper with family the girls' father showed up. He made it clear he wanted to speak to me in private. He then told me his daughter had said I had beaten her. Then I proceeded to tell him what had happened and what had taken place afterward. I definitely had paddled her rear. He also said he had asked some of the people and servers before talking to me. I told him I would apologize but please keep her away from me. He told me no need to apologize. He should have paddled her long before this she had lied to him and it wasn't the first time. We shook hands and I invited him to sit and have a meal with us. He thanked me but refused my invite. He said he was a little too upset to eat at this time. Word got out about what had happened. The men would look at me and smile and just chuckle.

Chuck mom Sue and Chum Were Doing the Town, mom and Sue doing the shopping Chuck and Chum Escorting Them. Chuck and Chum would leave to take care of some of their business things, then would come back to pick them up. We had a lot of invites to different homes. The father of the girl I had asked if I could Court invited us to dinner also. I felt good about this, would give mom and Sue Chum and Chuck a chance to meet the girl I was interested in. Wanted their opinions, respected their judgments. They were always sensible. The evening meal went well with a lot of laughter especially the stories that had to get out about the girl in my room. My chosen girl's father said any other man would have had no problem of bedding her. My answer was she was very immature and quite silly. Jan my chosen girl agreed. Then asked me if I would accompany her on a horseback ride she and a couple of girls had planned for in a few days, of course I agreed.

Next day went back to the blacksmith shop to enjoy the men and see all the new things that had been devised. A steam engine was being tried out. Sometimes during a dry season they loss waterpower, steam driven would supplement their power needs. After leaving the shop just wandered the streets. Learn to stay away from the side streets. They were throwing their garbage into the street hoping for big rainstorm to flush it away. The stench wasn't to my liking. The city was in a place where I would never live, the upper class lived quite comfortably. The middle class seem to get along quite well also. The lower-class just put up with whatever came their way. At times quite violent as I had found out with my excursions into the working part of the city. The blacksmith shop was part of this environment. To me the farm was the ideal place to live, I had enjoyed my life with the Indians. After my bride died everything seem to change. I would go back and visit but would not live with him again. Had enjoyed the trading forays with the chief and my Indian brother and an tracker friend I had made. Thinking on this part of my life it was one of the happiest times.

We had many invites to evening meals by other businessmen

A Past Life: as told by Brave Hawk

that Chuck and Chum were acquainted with. Two days to the horseback ride Jan had planned went by quickly. Went and got my filly and dog. The hostler had made good friends with my dog. He told me if I ever wanted to give him up he would take him in a heartbeat. I knew my dog stayed there because my filly was there and I told him to stay. I knew if my filly had not been there he would be out looking for me. Still could tell he liked the hostler very much. I still rode without a saddle just a blanket over my filly's back. Had other parts made up in front to carry my rifle in my bow. Had saddle type bags on her rump for other things I carried for longer trips. Wouldn't need those for a day's jaunt. Jan told me where we would meet. Just on one of the lesser roads leading out of the city. I had wandered the city to know exactly where she meant. It saved me a trip through the city and back tracking to the rode she had planned for her excursion. Got there early didn't mind waiting was a beautiful day. Wasn't long and Jan in her two friends and one of her girls boyfriends the other girls beau couldn't make it. Jan and one of the other girls were split skirts for riding. This was something that was frowned on by the older woman. One girl was riding side-saddle. She had chosen a very spirited horse. To me she didn't look as though she could handle him very well. We had no more than got started with her horse started to act up. She yanked on the reins making the horse rear up throwing her off. We made sure she was okay then went after her horse. The other girls' boyfriend finally caught up to the horse and grabbed the reins. The horse was still quite frisky. We led him back to where the girls were waiting. I made the decision, would ride the horse that had thrown the girl. She would ride my filly. My filly had never had a saddle tied on so it was a few minutes before she stopped high-stepping, calmed her down by talking to her in Indian. She seemed a lot more at ease with me talking to her in the Indian language. She settled down within a few minutes. The girl was in kind of skeptical about riding a horse that wasn't guided by rains. I told her she would follow me. She would sense you are a little apprehensive, she was very good with kids and others that were learning to ride. If they got mean and tried to beat her she would throw them off. They would not be able to get near her again. Took my bow and not any arrows and mounted bareback on the frisky horse. He tried to buck me off, I was used to this so didn't have much problem with staying on. Took my bow and gave him a sharp rap on the rump this got him heading down the road. When he started to slow down just gave him another sharp rap to keep him going I was going to tire him out completely. Finally I could tell he was getting winded pulled him to stop to wait for the others he had worked up a good lather. Was rubbing him down with handfuls of grass. Everyone showed up shortly. Jan shook her head, they didn't know how I had stayed on especially without a saddle. They were all amazed at my riding and then at my rubbing the horse down. They had thought I was going to beat the heck out of him. I told him he just needed a good run. He needed to be rubbed down, would walk him to help cool him down. Then let everyone go ahead I would follow. Took the horses reins and jogged alongside of the horse. Jan in the group are just walking the horses so I just went on by jogging alongside the horse, felt I was also in need of a good run after being in the city without any good exercise. I ran steady for a long time checking the horse to make sure he had cooled down and would be all right. This is something we had done when with the Indians. They could run all day and probably more. My tracking friend and Indian brothers wouldn't even look tired after a daylong run. I could do it but would be tired at the end of the day. They would laugh at me when I would just flop down took a while before getting accustomed to this. Wasn't long before I could keep up with them. Could out run them for a distance but couldn't keep the pace up and they would catch up and go by me. I learned to pace myself like they did and then could keep up. Jan rode up to my side and asked if I was getting tired, not yet was my answer. She said it wasn't but a couple of miles more. Just told her to lead the way and would follow. Jan finally pulled off a well-used trail. This went to a lake, there were some cabins some lean'tos establish on the lake shore. Jan said her father had one of them built. This is a nice set up. We then unpacked and let the horses roam the rest brought hobbles for their horses. Asked me if I was going to hobble my filly, my answer

A Past Life: as told by Brave Hawk

was no she had never been hobble she had a halter but never had a rein hooked to her mouth. Told him she would come to my whistle.

As we approach the door the cabin two men came out they surprised us. Jan wanted to know what they were doing the cabin was privately owned by her. They just smiled and stood in our way. Then Guy stepped forward he acted like he was going to tackle into them. I had been standing next to my filly so they had not noticed me, when I stepped forward they realize there was more than just one man. Just looking at them could see they were not expecting me. What I did notice one had a knife in his hand. When I stepped up with the other man they decided two against two wasn't to their advantage. They backed off and left down another trail. Then told the girls would be back in a few minutes. Went into the woods to get ahead of them the man his name Guy wanted to come along with me. I told him just in case there were others he best stay and protect the woman. I would not be gone long. I hit the trail quite a bit in front of them. They had stopped watch us unpacked. I was darn good at moving silently through the woods came up behind them, gave them a hell of a surprise when I grunted behind them. The older man still had the knife in his hand. Hadn't drawn my knife as yet, they looked at me then started to get belligerent. My next words were for the man with the knife, to drop it on the ground. He looked at me then he suddenly realized who I was, rumors and word had gotten out I was one dangerous person. Then told them I could track them anywhere. Best they leave if they came back and used the cabin again they would probably forfeit their life. I stepped into the woods motioning them to leave. The one bent to pick up the knife I told him to leave it. They both then left I followed for a ways to make sure they were not coming back. Then headed for the cabin they were worried about me asking what went on. Just told them wanted to make sure they left and would not ambush us when we had thought they were gone.

We had a good meal Jan in the girls were good cooks. The young man and I hit it off and we talked, he telling me what he did. He said he did a lot of running to keep fit. Said he couldn't have run anywhere as far as I had run running with the horse. I told him the Indians did this all the time. I was not up to my normal self, because of being in the city. He laughed and said he wished he could do what I had. He then asked me about my filly. I told him my filly wasn't used to a saddle I never used one. As long as I was close by she would tolerate the saddle. If she didn't like someone they would have a hard time staying on her back. When the girls were busy, I then had a serious talk about approaching someone like these two men. They were cowards but would take advantage of any situation. Told him would teach him what I had been taught, he readily agreed. Went and cut some alders to act as a knife and Tomahawk for a left-hand protection. He went into to tell the girls what we were going to do they wanted to watch. Then told them why you should have something in your left hand My tomahawk was for my left hand, also made sure to tell my new friend to always make sure to know if they were left-handed, it would change the fighting entirely. We sparred for a while, he was quite good showed him some of the twisting turns he could use by using his left hand to Ward off others blows and thrusts. He could make his own thrusts at the same time. Afterward we relaxed and talked about the city life and I about the farm and sawmill, blacksmith shop. They then asked if I thought these men would be back. I told them they were more than likely to be back after we left so don't leave anything of value. I then told Guy you should never approach men as he did without being ready. I was holding the knife he probably would've used. When they saw that there was two of us the odds then work in our favor so they back down. I then gave Guy the knife that the other man had left. He then asked me if I had done the other two men in. I laughed and said no I had never done anyone in only in self-defense. He then asked how in the world did I get his knife. Told Guy the man was so surprise when I stepped out in front of them he just dropped it. So figured it would be a good reminder of our trip to the lake.

Told Guy on the side these men would definitely be back

A Past Life: as told by Brave Hawk

after we left. I may come back and surprising them. He was all excited about the challenge and insisted he come with me. We had a leisurely ride back to the city. Guy and I made plans on our next excursion to the lake. Also Jan invited me to dinner, she said she wanted to show me off to her other friends. They were excited to meet me. The evening was planned in two days.

Next day Guy approached me and asked if we were going out to the lake, told him if we went better bring our rifles. These men may give us more trouble if we weren't armed. We got everything ready and I took my bow as I always like the way it made very little noise compared to a rifle. Guy looked my rifle over and like it very much, was one I had done up myself. Made to my liking, also worked very well. We packed a lunch and left for the lake took our time Guy asked about the bow. Took a little time to show him I was very efficient with a bow, very accurate at 50 to 75 yards. We headed up the trail and went only halfway and dismounted my dog was with us. He had been trained to be very quiet also. Guy thought he would probably start barking, I laughed and said he was an Indian dog and was very intelligent. He won't bark will give a light growl if he feels were being watched, or if anyone threatens us. Will only attack on my command. He also only understood the Indian language I spoke. He then said I can't wait till tomorrow evening for you to relate some of your Indian experiences. I guided Guy and myself through the woods to the cabin. Stopped at the opposite side of the main approach to the cabin. We waited for a short while watching the cabin. Didn't see any sign of movement as yet. My dog all the sudden gave a low growl. This is when one of the men came out of the cabin. I told Guy to get his rifle ready just in case. I would step out challenging him. Stepping into view he was surprised again to see me he then ducked back into the cabin yelling for his partner. Next was a rifle poking out of a window. I then dropped and rolled his shot missed me, but Guys shot took in in the head. He would not be shooting again. Told his buddy he had best come out or the same fate awaited him. Guy had thought that I had been hit the way I had dropped them rolled. Had relied on Guy to cover me and he did a good job. Guy then told me this was the second time he had shot someone. The other was in self-defense when an intruder at his home had tried to shoot him. He said I was ready for him and got off a better shot. The Intruders shot had missed his shot had done the intruder in. The boy in the cabin finally came out. He was almost crying. He figure we were going to take him back to the city to be locked up, that was not a good experience. Guy looked at me and shrugged his shoulders. We next made him bury his buddy and clean up the Gore in the cabin. I had a talk with Guy and told him to much of a hassle to bring the boy back. If he had not learned his lesson someone else would take care of him. We then marched him out to the main road and pointed him in the opposite direction we were headed. He then realized we were letting him go. He turned as he left surprise both of us. He thanked us many times with a slight bow. We told him we had no intentions of harming him or his partner but his partner brought it on himself. We had found another rifle loaded and ready to go next to him. We knew he had meant to do someone in if they caught him at the cabin again. He agreed and said he shouldn't have been chumming with him. We then shared some of our food and coin and send him on his way. Guy and myself hope he would learn and do better for himself Guy asked me if we should relate this to the police. I said no it was finished as far as I was concerned, he agreed wholeheartedly. The police at times got carried away with their investigation. A few were like the one that had been done in by someone and found in the river with his skull caved in.

Guy asked if he could tell his friends about our excursion, that was fine with me. We should both agree that if the police should ask us, our story should be just as it happened. Telling the truth we wouldn't have to deny anything. The authorities had enough to do without investigating a story. Back to the stable and brush my filly down and did the same for my dog. The hostler was amazed at my dog staying within my filly. He said the dog would go out and relieve himself would stay out for a while as though waiting for me to show up. He told me he had made friends with him. No one else

A Past Life: as told by Brave Hawk

could get near him or my filly. One of the other hands had tried to get near my filly and no way was my dog going let him. So he's the one that had taken care of both my filly and my dog. My dog would even let him brush him. I told him my dog knows you are trustworthy person.

Next morning had breakfast with the family. Chuck and Chum mom and Sue were enjoying the city. They had rounded up a lot of cloth, cotton, linen and some very fine wool. They were really excited about their findings, also were having a wonderful time at all the invites we were getting. When they had gone without me, everyone asked where I was. I didn't always enjoy the evening too many questions for me to try to answer. Sometimes I would get the impression they didn't believe my stories. I would get exasperated about some of the stupid questions and remarks. Everyone was invited out to dinner that evening. Mom asked if I was going, told of her Jan had invited me to a get together with her friends. Mom was thrilled that I was seeing Jan. Aunt Sue gave me a nod and knowing smile. She took me aside and told me she and Jan had talked for quite some time. Jan had asked if what I had related was true or just a made up story. Chum had told her that one thing I didn't do was lie or make up stories. What was said was true, also was leaving out a lot of the things that had happened and most wouldn't believe. Chum said have me take my shirt off and the scars of my chest and side would confirm to the truth of my stories. Chum said how I had survived was just plain good fortune. She then said to Jan ask me to speak in the Indian language. Chum said I was fluent in their language. The only time I spoke Indian was to my dog, my filly seem to understand both.

Next morning went back up to the blacksmith shop. Stopped at the hostlers and got my dog to come with me, he never showed much sign of excitement like other dogs would. Could tell he was always glad to see me, would just come to me and sit at my side. My hostler friend told me if I ever wanted to get rid of my dog he would take him in a heartbeat. I had the other men come over and I introduced him to my dog. This way he would know they were also friends. He would then let them approach him and my filly, they all got a charge out of the dog that would know to make friends when I introduced them to him. Told them didn't want any harm to come to them or him. Then he invited all out to lunch at the tavern close by. Someone would have to stay behind to keep track of things, always someone wanted a horse taking care of. Told him I would make it up to him. Would take him out for lunch the next stop. Just happened that my hostler friend who was caring for my filly and dog, had volunteered to stay and take care of things. We went to the tavern and everyone had a good lunch most had beer with their meal. I drank a glass of wine. After the meal went to the blacksmith shop wanted to see how the steam engine was doing. The men all welcome me, the steam engine had been set up and they had it running a few times. Seems like it was going to work out well for them.

After a leisurely walk back up to the better part of town, just felt I had to have a good run. Miss my Indian friends we had always ran every day we would run alongside of our horse just for the pleasure running. My trapper friend and Indian brother and myself could run all day and not seem tired. I could do this but would be tired at the end of the day. We, that is my dog and me found a path that look like a good place for a run. Took off up the path with my dog ahead and sometime behind me. Had not gone too far when we were approached by someone on horseback. They turned the horse sideways and on the path to stop me. He then told me were trespassing, I then apologize, told him that it had looked like a good path to take a long run-on. Didn't realize that we were trespassing wouldn't have chosen the path if I had known. He looked at me in a kind of questioning way, then asked who I was. Told him I was visiting the city with family, he got off his horse and offered his hand to me. He then apologize saying he had not recognize meat first. We visited for a while just on general things. He finally introduced himself, I knew he was Jan's father. He said he had heard a lot of stories. My answer was they always get

A Past Life: as told by Brave Hawk

exaggerated he laughed and knew what I meant. He said I knew Jan was having a surprise party this evening. I then told him I was invited. He laughed again and said that I was her surprise. She hadn't told him about what her surprise was. He then said let's surprise her with you showing up now. I told him I was in my old clothes and would need to bathe and change first. He understood and said you do look different in your workaday outfit. I didn't recognize you at first, then he asked me if all the details about me were true. My answer again was everything gets exaggerated. He just nodded, will see you this evening. Told me how to get to his home the back way. He then said let's surprise Jan by your coming into the back door and kitchen. I will wait till everyone is there and make them wait a little, then will bring you out and say sorry we were talking got carried away in the kitchen. He then said Jan will be a little put out, he wasn't supposed to know or interfere. He said he enjoyed a little prank once in a while himself. He would make it right with Jan if she got to upset. He said she was a heck of a good girl and he doubted if she would be upset.

That evening showed up in my best buckskin clothes always with my knife on my shoulder, Tomahawk on my left hip. Mom and Sue wanted me to leave my knife and Tomahawk at the inn. Told them just felt naked without them. Would remove them when I got to their place for supper.

As Jan's father had asked me to come to the back way he would be there to meet me. We then went into the kitchen and sat with the cook and maids Jan's father had a good rapport with his help. He also stated Jan was also a very good cook. She had got into the kitchen to do the her thing. The cook had thought she didn't approve of his cooking. She went to him and apologize telling him she and her dad were very pleased with him and his cooking. She just wanted to learn herself and would appreciate any advice he gave her. Jan apologize again. After that they got along real well. They had two maids to do the pickup and cleaning .Jan's guests began to arrive. Her father peeking out to see how many had arrived. Jan was at the door greeting them, most were young folks our age. Guy was one of the guests. When Jan's dad had decided no more were coming he had me step out and just stand leaning on the door jam. He also insisted I leave my knife and my Tomahawk on, I wanted to leave them in the kitchen. He said just for effect, wanted to see Jan's face when she spotted me. Everyone had been watching the front door expected me to show any time. One of the girls turned around and I was standing very close, she let out a squeal that even made me jump. I could hear Jan's father laughing in the kitchen. Janet first looked a little upset. Then she had big grin. Began to introduce me to her friends all seem quite excited about my entrance. How did I get in without anyone seeing me. I said I just walked in and stood by the door didn't understand how no one had even notice me. Jan before we sat down to supper took me aside and said dad put you up to this, I had to agree. Jan's reply was well I was supposed to surprise everyone but dad did a better job. He then said everyone will remember this evening. I said before I sit down would shed my knife and Tomahawk. Jan laughed and said another little touch of dads, he had you leave them on, just shrugged my shoulders. Any other girl would be very upset but not Jan all she had to say was wish she had thought of it herself. The evening went very well, didn't relate any stories or information only when asked. Jan asked me if I would speak in Indian. I know no one would understand what I was saying. She then said you could tell us what you said. I finally agreed, Jan said we would wait till little later in the evening. I let Jan know that the Arapahoe language was very hard to speak. Even now don't always get it quite right. When I did speak I then translated then told them I was thanking them for coming and that the food was much better than dog, when I related to what was said they had a good laugh about the dog part. All wanted to know how in the world I was able to learn the language. Then related if you live with them and that was all that was spoken doesn't take long to learn. There was the girls asked if I had killed a lot of Indians. My answer was no. Of course they had heard about my fight with the two men I had done in when I first got to the city. She started to question me about that, Jan seeing how uncomfortable she was

A Past Life: as told by Brave Hawk

making me and again came to my rescue and said we had to go to the front door everyone was leaving. Everyone complimented me on my buckskin outfit, it was my best Indian outfit the Indian woman had made for me it was very elaborate. My first wedding outfit was even more elaborate. Beads and ermine tales and other things. They wondered why I had not worn that outfit. I had not worn it since Running Deer had crossed over. She was the only woman I had ever known. None had appealed to me since until I met Jan. Jan and her father asked me to stay the night. I told them Mom Sue Chum and Chuck would be expecting me. They would want to know how the evening went. I was glad the girl I had paddled wasn't there. Jan said she had invited her but was turned down. Jan came out to the stables with me, my dog just seemed to know Jan went to her and sat at her feet. Jan my dog is abandoning me for you. She just said I have a good rappore with animals didn't offer to kiss her, Jan had other ideas and gave me a real hard kiss after my filly bump me into her looking for attention. I was flabbergasted and tongue-tied. I knew that she was to be my new wife. I asked her as soon as I could get my tongue to say something if she would marry me. Her answer was you were for me the first time I had seen you at the party that she had rescued me from the giggling girls. I went back to the inn seems like I was floating on air. When I entered the inn everyone was up and waiting for me. Mom and Sue could see I was very excited. Mom looked at me and said you're going to marry Jan, Sue nodded in agreement, how the heck did they know. They just said they knew we should be together. We were scheduled to leave the city in two days, mom and Sue said they would invite Jan back to our farm. I was elated, then asked would it be all right if I invited a friend and his gal also. Mom and Sue agreed. We had plenty of rooms after Chuck and Chum had expanded the old home the sawmill made it easy to build and still make a good profit from the mill.

Met Jan the next day for lunch. Then asked if she and her girlfriend and Guy would like to accompany me and my family back to our home I told her it was nothing like the city but was quite comfortable. Jan told me she would ask Guy and see if he could go. He and his father had a business in the city of which was doing quite well. Told mom and Sue they agreed to postpone leaving for another day. Jan invited me for supper with her father. I decided to ask her father for Jan's hand in marriage that evening. After the meal out of earshot of Jan, I asked her father if he had any objections to my proposal. His reply was his only objection if I had not asked Jan already. I laughed and told him I already had. He just laughed and said he could see how much she really cared for me. Jan had not been interested in very many gentlemen. They were as she had told her father they were too much city. They had no other outlook which was monotonous for her. He said he could see the change in Jan right away. She told her dad about me paddling one of the girls and sending her home in her carriage. She then told her dad if I showed any interest, she wouldn't be pushing me away. Jan sure showed me this last night. Jan's father then told me he would have all the wedding arrangement made when we came back from our trip to the farm. The wagon was set up so the woman could sleep fairly comfortable. This wagon was tarp covered. Mom and Sue rode horses like the rest of us saying riding was a touch more enjoyable then bouncing in the wagon. Chuck Chum Guy and myself slept outside. We were prepared for wet weather with extra tarps attached to the side of the wagons. We had made cots that were folded and mounted under the wagon. With all of cloth and the other merchandise, just barely enough room for the woman to sleep, they said they would make do.

We had been on other trips just for enjoyment that had been a lot rougher then this trip. On the way back to the farm we had only one day of rain and not any hard downpours or storms when we arrived at the farm everyone settled in quite well. They were quite surprised at how well mom and Aunt Sue had done the house. The house looked as good as any in the city houses we had been in. Wanted to show Jan and my friends Guy and his girl the sawmill and barn and hoped the old mule was still around. To my surprise my dog had gone into the pasture and here came the mule behind

A Past Life: as told by Brave Hawk

my dog. The mule came and greeted me with a lot of snuffing. I had to go out and get a brush and brush him down. He was getting quite old his partner had already crossed over. I couldn't get over how he still recognize me being gone for so long a stretch of time. Jan was fascinated by the old Guy. I told her that the mules put up with me when I was a lot younger. Father had thought at 1st they might stomp me. They put up with all my somersaults and often landing on their backs. Even my going under their bellies didn't faze them. Only a few men could handle them. If they didn't like someone they had to be darned careful they didn't get stomped on or bitten. Jan could see I really love this old mule. When the other mule had gotten sick, mom and Sue tried to nurse him back to health but it was his time to go. So they retired the other mule and just left him to enjoy the pasture life. My dog came and would sit by me and the mule while I was grooming him. I then groomed my dog. He wasn't crazy about being groomed but would put up with it. Jan asked if my dog ever barked. Told her I had never heard him bark but make a little woofing sound as a warning, a growl if it was something he didn't trust

Jan wanted to know how I had come by the dog. She could see how very attached he was to me. Then related how we, that is my Indian friends went looking to trade for dogs. We had heard about another tribe that had a lot of dogs. We found they were about 4 to 6 months old. We had picked four out of one litter two out of another. One of them came over and sat by my feet, where ever I moved he would come and sit by me. Then told her how the other sub chief had said he wouldn't include him in the trade. My chief and Indian brothers bristled up and said the trade was already done we were leaving with the dogs including the one that had adopted me. Then the sub chief said they would kill the dog before we left his village. My trapper friends' chief and my brother all had knocked arrows in their bows and told him his life would be the only one that would be killed. He decided to back down right away after seeing arrows would be loosed at him. We then backed out of the village very cautiously. The chief and my trapper friend Gonacheaw knew that the other chief would try something. They had both had a good idea where he would try this. We only had three horses amongst us at the time. So we weren't moving very fast because of the dogs. One of the trappers and came back in and said they were moving out to set up their ambush in front of us. My brother and myself had went to the other side checking for any one moving around us. The chief sent two of our men out front on the run to get into position to ambush them. Our ambush was successful they had killed two of the four that had planned on ambushing us. We now had two more horses. The other chief and the other had escaped. We knew that this would be one sub chief we would have to keep an eye on. My dog had stayed by my side ever since. He's very well behaved and knew what I wanted him to do he would stay with my filly if I told him to stay.

Guy and his gal came and joined Jan in me I asked if they would like to see the sawmill, there have been a lot of improvements. They were also very surprised at the water coming into the house by Cedar pipes Chum Chuck and I had devised and piped the spring water into the kitchen even the valve was wood more like a tapered plug the sink also drained to the outside. This was quite convenient, we now had a cook in the main kitchen. Mom and Sue were able to spend a lot more time in their herb garden and a lot of flowers. When the biting flies were bad mom and Sue had come up with herb repellent that worked real well and was not offensive to the nose.

Next day Guy and his gal Bess Jan and I went up to the sawmill. Still running smoothly Chuck and Chum had made quite a few improvements including a lathe to turnout pillars and posts. The men all welcomed us and explain to the girls what was going on. There was always a call for lumber. We then enjoyed a picnic lunch I then said would like to go into the village and visit with my blacksmith friends. That afternoon we all went to see the blacksmith's we were all welcomed and were served tea and some other breads of some kind and were very good .They had to tell

A Past Life: as told by Brave Hawk

my friends about some of my exploits when I was younger. Had to tell them about my meeting the bully that had came to town and left much the worse. Also how no one could beat me in a race of any kind. Also, Chum and I had out shot everyone. Spent a nice afternoon, then headed back to the farm. They didn't relate about the hanging that had taken place to my relief.

We got back to the farm supper was almost ready. We all sat down enjoyed a glass of wine our maid came out to do the serving this was new to me. Mom and Sue just rolled their eyes and grinned. The maid was a heck of a good worker, she didn't have any family. Mom and Sue tried to find out but she said they were all gone that was all the information she gave. The meal was very good, the cook was also very good. Had to go to the kitchen and complement the cook on his meal. He hadn't expected that of me but was very pleased. The maid was a little afraid of me because I carried my knife and Tomahawk whenever I left the house. Started to leave the Tomahawk hanging on the clothes pegs. Could tell she was afraid of me. I asked Jan to intercede for me I didn't like to have anyone afraid of me. Jan said she would find a way to catch her off guard and would have a chat. Jan later that evening got me to go into the kitchen with her. Our maid was sitting in having her supper. We surprised her and she started to get up and Jan said just came in to visit with you and the cook. We could see that she was still quite apprehensive. We got to chatting took a while but she finally opened up to Jan we talked about general things how Jan and I were engaged to marry, we would be married in the city I asked if she would like to come this took her by surprise. She said to me you would invite me to your wedding. Jan answered for me and said of course. She declined but could see she was very much relaxed. She then told us she had come from the city to hide from her husband he was a drinker and got very mean. She just up and left him. Didn't have any children so wasn't hard to leave him. Going back to the city he would probably find her. But it was very nice to be invited to your wedding .Guy had also proposed to his girl and she had also accepted .They then came to Jan and me and asked if it could be a double ceremony. Jan and I were more than willing. I found Guy to be an honest and trustworthy fellow. Was glad to have them for a friend. Jan had originally introduced her friend Bess to Guy. I found that Jan was a childhood friend with her girlfriend Bess, Guy had been courting other girls but found most not to his liking until introduced to Jan's friend Bess. Things blossomed from there.

Talked with Chum about the small lake we had enjoyed when we were younger he said he had not been up there for a while he and Chuck had made a large lean to the fishing was still really good. So asked Guy best and Jan if they would be up to an outing at the lake, they were all for it. Chuck then told me had laid claim to the land and lake was included in the survey our land now was quite extensive next day we decide to walk in and take one horse as a pack animal to carry all our essentials. The bugs weren't too bad with mom and Sue's bug repellent made the trip enjoyable. The lean to to was quite elaborate, enclosed except for the front. We had brought netting as screen to keep the night time bugs and skeeters out. Even had a fireplace at the back wall. The lean-to was built near a spring so the water was good. The lake water would have been also potable. We unpacked and got set up. Found a wooden boat Chum had told us about we flip the boat right side up and backed away in a hurry a skunk was underneath. No one got sprayed the skunk then ambled over and went under the lean to. We weren't about to disturb him any further. Guy had pulled the boat to the lake. The boat was made just for two people the girls said for us to go try to catch some fish. They would finish setting up the camp. We were out on the lake in a short time we had caught enough fish for both supper and breakfast. We came back into shore and cleaned the fish, girls had got everything ready for supper. Mom and Sue had packed a bottle of wine in with the food. Guy and I went to the lake to wash up after cleaning the fish. I pulled my shirt and undershirt off and proceeded to wash. Guy had done the same, Guy looked at me with an odd look. He didn't say anything so I let it pass. We got back to the lean to the girls had the wine open and were waiting for us. We then enjoyed the wine, Jan and Bess cooked the fish we all sat with

A Past Life: as told by Brave Hawk

our legs hanging out of the entrance of the lean to plates on our laps Guy surprised me by asking how I got the scars on my side and arm and my chest. I then chuckled and said I wondered why you had a puzzled look when we were washing up and told them it was a bear and a Tomahawk but didn't elaborate. We ate our meal and talked about our coming weddings we were all quite excited. Before the evening was over Jan and Bess said are you going to tell us about the scars. I just grinned and said I thought I had. Bess said oh Bird we wanted to know how and what happened. So related what had came about and how fortunate to have survived both times. With a fire going and the netting we had put up it was quite cozy in the lean to the girls curled up on one side and Guy and I on the other. The morning breakfast was also very good eggs and fried meat and some fish. My mom and father didn't care for pork rarely had it. Mom had told me that a couple of the family had died from eating pork. We had food that had been stored in the spring. We're living like kings so Guy and Bess remarked. Our three days went by very fast, returned to the farm

That evening the girls went early to our bathhouse room. We had made a room with a tub. Had a fire going and a metal fireplace Chuck had made. Had large kettles for hot water. The girls couldn't get over how pleasant it was to soak in a tub of hot water. The whole family enjoyed the tub and the hot water. The girls bathed at the lake but was quite cold so was a quick bath. Had to laugh when mom took me aside and said these are not Indian girls you should be a gentleman. My answer was mom I have too much respect and love for Jan to try anything stupid. Could see mom was relieved she said she and Aunt Sue were very happy for me

Jan was an outdoors person. She told mom and Sue how she liked the farm and was amazed at their Herb garden. One can learn a lot more here. Almost time to head back to the city. Mom asked me if I was going to have a tailor-made suit for my wedding. My answer was I've worn buckskin as long as I can remember now so will continue to do the same. Dug out my original first wedding outfit. This was a very elaborate Indian outfits the woman from the tribe had made me. This was a very happy time in my life and this would bring back the happiness for me. mom and Sue agreed that it was more than appropriate.

Time to leave for the city, packed the horses started early. We made good time and were back in the city in an early afternoon. I went to the inn where we all had stayed was going to make arrangements to stay. Jan insisted I go home with her and stay at her father's house. Guy spoke up and said is Bird going to stay with you till were married. Jan agree she then asked Bess if she would stay with her Bess readily agreed they had been together since childhood and had always got along well. Jan said she knew her dad would have supper ready for us, so we had better come for supper. Jan's father had made all the arrangements and planed a party for both Jan and Bess. Jan's father had gotten together with Bess' father and both had invited all their friends. I had thought about what mom had said about a suit. So asked Jan if it would offend her if I wore my buckskin outfit she was more than glad to have me wear it. I like it because you are an outdoors man. She also commented that if anyone didn't like it so be it. The outfit was well made by loving hands. Made me feel good and relieved that Jan was so open-minded found her father was a same way.

The double wedding went off without any problems. My outfit stunned a lot of the people. I got comments that they had never seen a nicer-looking buckskin outfit before. Most tried to get me to drink more of the hard liquor that was being doled out. One glass of wine was my limit. Just didn't like my senses dulled. Seen too many men drunk and had no intention of doing the same. Told Jan that when it came to dancing was not very good. She just got me out on the floor and I managed not to make a fool of myself. We were staying at the house, we would be using Jan's bedroom. Our honeymoon was going back to the farm and back to the lake for a while. Jan had planned it with Bess and they were all for it Guy had also been told and he was also for it. As the evening progressed made

A Past Life: as told by Brave Hawk

the rounds to try to speak a little to everyone Jan at my side most of the time. One man kept giving me a sour look. Didn't bother trying to approach him. Would find Guy and asked him who he was. Guy knew right off, he said he had courted Jan they had went to dinner and Jan had not went with him again even though he had asked numerous times. Everything went well all were having a good time. As Jan and I headed back toward the kitchen this man's stepped over and grab Jan's arm. He made a big mistake by doing so had been keeping an eye on him and expected some kind of confrontation. Thought it would be me. Just stepped over and grabbed him by the throat and forced him back into the kitchen punched him in his solar plexus he was done in and moaning. Except for Jan and the people in the kitchen nobody had seen anything I believe he was trying to make a stir about our wedding hoping to spoil the evening. Still holding him by the throat walked him out backwards out the back door. Went out the door let go and he fell to his hands and knees I waited for him to catch his breath. Then let him know that he was a dead man if he ever tried anything again. One of the servants had went after Jan's father, Jan was just behind me. I asked if she was okay she said she was fine I could tell she was upset Jan's father showed up and had the stable boys haul this man off. Went back into the kitchen and Jan said to me he wasn't a boyfriend. I said I could see that he was just a mean blanket y-blank. Jan's father had not liked him either Jan said he had asked her out for dinner and had went the one time and found he was no gentleman. She had turned down all the advances after that. Jan asked me if I was upset over this my answer was not with you. This man would have been dead if he had been out in the Indian territory. I don't need the police on my neck, other than that I would have rung his neck.

Jan said I have had other suitors but they were all gentlemen. I just didn't connect with anyone tell you came along. Jan's father knew who he was and said he worked for some company in the city. He hadn't been invited to the wedding reception just came. Jan's father was also upset and he told me he would see this man didn't come around again. I didn't know what he had planned, had other things on my mind. Everyone left we headed up to Jan's room it was done up special. I decided the first night we would not make love let things calm down and just enjoy each other. We were both quite tired from the day's events, so we just talked, then crawled into bed held each other and fell asleep. Jan woke up first and headed for the bathing room. The maids had seen that the water was hot. She bathed that I went in and also bathed. Then we went back to bed and made love. We were both clumsy and did a lot of giggling. Jan said she thought I would be more aggressive and experience. I told her had known only one girl and she was my Indian wife. Jan was also a virgin she laughed when I said I was almost a virgin. Guy and Bess had stayed the night also. Jan said let's go barge in on them, I didn't think it a good idea but went along anyway. They were up also and were getting dressed when Jan and I barged in. Bess said she knew Jan would not be able to resist barging in. They were prepared, we were still in our night wear. We had not expected this but the maids came up and served us breakfast. We planned our honeymoon back at the farm and at the lake. Bess and Guy were included in our and their honeymoon. I found Guy to be an excellent companion. Although he was born in the city he was an excellent outdoors-man. He enjoyed the hunting and the woods. Had to tell him about my Indian friends, brother chief and the tracker Gonacheaw. Had to tell him how exceptional a tracker Gonacheaw was. I told him he could track anyone, even on bare rock. He would always comment, I was the only one he hadn't been able to track after escaping. He had never questioned me about it. I have yet to volunteer any information. We became very good friends. Anytime our chief decided on a hunt or any other escapade, he was always the one who made the plans of course with all our input. Guy said at first he thought I was putting on a very good act, after getting to know me, he then knew better. I suggested we Jan, Bess included could make a trip out West some time to our trading post and also meet my Indian friends.

Guy said he would have to get his business in order and then would be able to go. We would ask the girls later if they would be

A Past Life: as told by Brave Hawk

up to this kind of a trip. First we had our honeymoon to enjoy.

We stayed in the city for a few days, receiving compliments and good wishes from Jan, Bess, Guys friends. We then packed up and headed for the farm. We had a pleasant trip, mom and Sue were expecting us and had planned a party for us. We had all the help including a sawmill hands, everyone had a good meal and a good time, different games were played, cards and some dice games were also enjoyed. Just one really pleasant evening. Seemed good to have such a wonderful family and good friends, Jan, Bess and Guy fit in just like family. Everyone commented on Jan's hair, it wasn't blonde but was very light also the way she had done it up for the get-together. Bess was also an outstanding girl with red hair. We loafed around the farm for a day or two before heading to the lake. Chuck and Chum knew of our plans to stay at the lean to. They had gone and made improvements for us. They had actually made it a little larger and made a kitchen and a room. What a surprise we got there. We were thankful for the improvements, especially after hard rain and thunderstorms hit while there. First few days we stayed inside playing card games, we also liked to read and had packed books in with us. So we had a good time despite the weather. Wasn't long before the sun was out, Jan I went out on the lake the fish. We again had good fortune and caught enough speckles for supper and breakfasts. The time just seemed to fly by, we made love even in the woods chuckled about it. Guy and Bess we imagine did the same. I would sit and think how fortunate I was to have two beautiful woman in my life again. Couldn't see how it could get any better.

Guy had to be back in the city to check on his and his father's business. He said he was trying to find a good and honest bookkeeper, also a good manager. He said he had someone in mind for both positions. Had to check out their credentials. Then he and Bess would accompany Jan and I out to meet my Indian family as I called them.

Wanted to make more plans for the sawmill and to make some

more additions. Maybe even a steam engine. Plan on a planer but had to perfect the speed to rotate a knives fast enough and have enough power without stalling. Jan was also interested in of all the machinery. She caught on to the workings very quickly. Also had input that was very helpful making a few changes would make it not only more efficient but also much easier to handle the lumber.

Mill wasn't anything like when Chum and I first started. Many improvements a circular saw for the smaller logs, larger logs were still sawed with a straight blade. Then the circular saw was used to finish into usable lumber. Jan and I were at the sawmill a lot of the time, she enjoyed the machinery and the gang of men and boys as much as I did. Chuck and Chum had hired a foreman who was very well-liked. He wouldn't put up with any slackers but would give breaks when needed. We also insisted on a full hour for noon lunch. Was hard to believe how far the mill had progressed. The water from the brook we had tapped into was more than adequate to run the mill. There were now three waterwheels to run the difference saws and the new planer we had devised. Once the kinks were worked out of the planer it worked quite well. Jan and I enjoyed the plans and figuring out what had to be done to get the planer working properly. A lot of adjustments and finally we were putting out smooth boards.

Jan and I headed back to the city to check on Guy and Bess. We were invited to Guys father's house for evening meal. We stayed with Jan's father and I found him to be an enjoyable companion. He also told me the one we had thrown out of the house at the time of our wedding was watching the house. He said watch for trouble from this Guy also stated he thought this Guy was crazy. I said I never look for trouble but it always seems to find me. When Jan and I left for dinner with Guy and Bess I knew he was following. If not him he had hired a couple of others to follow us. My dog also seem to know, was amazed at the senses dog of mine had. He and my tracker friend Gonacheaw had this sense. My senses were keen because of Gonacheaw's teaching. I was not as good as he and the

A Past Life: As Told by Brave Hawk

other trackers were. He always complimented me telling me I was as good as he, I knew better. Was pleased with his compliments.

Guys' father was also very pleasant. Her mother more than welcomed Jan and I into their home. She was thrilled with Guy's choice of Bess for a wife. We enjoyed the meal and Guy and Bess invited us to go and see his business the next day. Jan and I were both delighted to go. We left early for Jan's dad's house. We had just got started when two horsemen cut us off. My dog charge for the horses and the horse through one of the rider's off. I call my dog back and he settled by my horse still on the alert. The other man was the one we had thrown out of the house on our wedding evening. He started yelling and said he was challenging me to a duel. He would send his emissary to the house. The other man picked himself up and went to collect his horse and had a hard time catching him. We waited till they left, then proceeded to Jan's home. When we got there Jan related to her father what had happened. She wanted to leave the city right away. I told her I had met up with a lot more dangerous people than this man. That evening his emissary showed up., with a brace of pistols with him I told him my choice of weapons was a bow and arrow at 50 yards. He was the Challenger, I made the weapons choice. I thought he would back down on this challenge. His emissary had came back and accepted and even had chosen a place. I declined his place and told him would let him know where to meet. His emissary finally came back and agreed. I didn't want any surprises from his side. He was just crazy enough to try to have someone ambush me ,by choosing my location would have Jan's father's help in making sure no one was hiding to ambush us. I came to the conclusion I would have to probably do this man in or could expect a lot of problems from him in the future.

We had a leisurely day doing a lot of walking on her father's estate he had a beautiful apple orchard and grapevines were well kept up. His gardens were also well cared for. Sure was nice to have the funds to be able to keep up this estate. After talking to Jan's father found that the produce from his gardens and orchards paid the help and made him a good profit. Went back to Guys in Bess for another meal. Made plans to go with a Guy and Bess and his father to see his business. The business was textile they had a lot of woman and men sewing and weaving materials. They made some very fancy clothes catering to a lot of the upper class. Also made a lot of clothes for the working class. Could see it was a going concern Guy and his father figured they had a couple of good men to oversee the work and also the sales. I could see this was a good money maker. Guys dad was very pleasant, someone told him about the dual coming up. He told me he knew this man he was considered very dangerous. He was not to be trusted so keep your eye on him to try and pull off some kind of trick. His father had crossed over and left him money. There was questions on how his father had died no proof could be found of any wrongdoing. Everyone was surprised his father had seemed in good health. I then told Guys dad that Jan's father had staked out the place where it was to take place. I had thought he would have backed out.

Had not much experience with bow and arrow. Bess' father told me he will pull something off so watch him. He has the money to hire thugs.

The day came for the dual and I asked Jan not to come. Her dad would be with me and some of the workers would be keep an eye out for any tricks on the field. No one was going to be able to sneak in on either end of the field. Everything was set, we had a flagman who would drop the flag when we were to shoot. We then walked back to our positions. Had my bow and knocked an arrow and was ready, watching him all the time. Seeing another man come out from the side to meet him at his spot. I knew something wasn't quite right. So instead of watching the flagman watched him. The flagman had raised the flag when I saw my opponent raise a rifle. I then drew back my arrow and letting go as a saw the flash of the rifle. The slug crease my ribs on my right side knocking me back and the wind out of me for a few seconds. Looked up and could see my opponent on the ground. Jan came running out she knew I had been hit. I had already knocked another arrow just in case someone else was going to take another shot at me. His companions were just standing over the top of him. The flagman came up to me and apologized. He said he should have suspected this man. I then went walking up to see if he was going to get up. I was quite sure I had hit him in the chest with my arrow. My arrow had went clean through his chest with a feathers still showing. The arrow had gone to his heart. We kept an eye on his two companions, they said he had told them it was rifles. Both were amazed at me doing him in with a bow,

I had turned when I drew my arrow back this is what save me from a punctured lung. Jan spoke up and said he almost did my husband in pointing to my side could then see the blood where the ball had hit me. I was thankful that it didn't break any ribs. His companion didn't know what to do. He had hired them to just be with him. Told him if he had any coin in his pocket they were welcome to it .I just wanted my arrow. Jan was insistent I head back to the house for patching up. When I arrived went into the kitchen with Jan and her dad. One of the maids was good at healing so she cleaned the gash and put some kind of Herb on it and wrapped cloth around my rib cage to hold everything in place. Jan's father said how you stayed on your feet he would never know.

When the ball had hit me I had stepped back a couple of feet and had doubled up some. Jan and her father knew I was hit. Jan had thought it was a lot worse than what it was. We were all thankful it wasn't any worse. I believe when I released my arrow I had turned just enough to have the ball wrapped me in the ribs. Pulling the bow back to shoot turned just enough to have the ball almost miss. We found out later that this Guy was an excellent shot. That afternoon one of the men brought my arrow back. He apologizes said he needed the money but didn't realize what was going on. He said this man had challenge others and they all had ignored him.

Jan treated me like a baby wanting to wait on me hand and foot. We had been invited to sup with Guy and Bess' mom and dad and Jan's father. Jan had wanted to cancel, I just told Jan I wasn't hurting that much and would enjoy going. So we ended up going for the meal. Couldn't believe the stories, just from early morning to that night. The story was I was shot in the chest and was still able to shoot an arrow and do the other man in. Bess' father had not expected us for dinner after hearing the story. They had spread the story that they didn't think I would live through the night. When we showed up for dinner he was aghast at first. Then Jan told him I definitely had been shot. She said she thought she was going to faint when she see me stagger back a few pace, then catch myself. Jan said she had not seen me shoot the arrow was watching the other man. Glad I had seen him raise the rifle. This had given me the chance to let my arrow fly. How thankful I was to my Indian friends with whom had taught me how to use the bow. Took a lot of practice to be real good with it. The maid that had patched me up also had seen my other scars. She also had added to the story that I must have survived a lot of fights. Told Jan and Bess' father had turned to draw my arrow back and believe this is what save me from getting the ball through the lung. To the men seeing the blood coming out of my shirt it looked like it had went into my chest. They had told everyone I was one tough person to be able to walk around with a ball in my chest. All I had to say was I just hope not to run into any more crazy people. The police officer was taken care of for me. I know the blacksmith had got rid of him. Then his father had died from heart failure after confronting me and accused me of his death. Made up my mind not to live in the city, the farm sawmill and our trading was more than enough to keep us busy. After dinner, Jan asked Guy and Bess if they were still interested in our planed excursion to meet my Indian family. Guy and Bess were all for it. Guy had talked it over with his father and he had said he would go himself if he were younger. He told Guy he had hired a good man and he could take care of the other end of the business. This would be a good experience for Guy, get the adventure and traveling out of his system. Jan's father agreed and also said if he

A Past Life: as told by Brave Hawk

was younger he would also go. I told Jan and Bess it would be hard going at times. Just the pleasure of seeing different land was well worth the hardships we would encounter.

Had sore ribs for a while but was thankful none were broken. Wasn't long and it scabbed over and healed. Would leave another scar now on my right side. Jan and I walked and sometimes ran we also rode our horses. I was getting restless to be back at the farm. I asked Jan if she would miss the city. Her answer was wherever you are I will be happy, felt darn good with that answer. Jan made sure I was well healed before heading back to the farm. We went and seen Guy and Bess before leaving to say our goodbyes. Both asked about going West to meet my Indian family. Told them it was too late in the season to make the trip. Would make plans for early next summer. Told him sometime spring brought heavy flooding. Good times to travels early summer and fall. Left that day before noon saying our goodbyes to others that we had befriended.

The trip went well without a hitch. Found new taverns had sprung up, Jan asked if I had ever stayed in one. Told her didn't like the bugs that accompanied these places and sometimes the clientele got real rowdy. A lot of drinking and occasionally fights. I just enjoyed the outdoors too much to sleep in such a wretched place. If the tavern was full you are expected to share the bed. It's not like the inns in the city. The better ones were clean but you also paid for the extra service.

Mom and Sue were glad to see us. They had carpenters in and made a room over just for us. A lot of expansion since I was a child. Everything seemed to be going quite well. Mom and Sue did well with the herb garden, also they were making clothes. So many things had changed over the last few years. We were doing well with the sawmill, trading post and the farm goods. Next morning made the sawmill our first visit they had some problem but Chum and Chuck Had Ironed Them out. Mostly our power system always needed repair.

Next day into the village to see what was up at the smithy's. Again we were more than welcome. The men had new apprentices who now were able to do a lot of the work easing up on our two blacksmith. Spent a few hours with them and their wives. They heard about my newest escapade and wanted to hear all about it. Just told them I had a dual and as they could see I survive. Jan gave me disgusted look. She said if you won't tell them I will. So she started at the beginning where we had thrown this man out at our wedding. Relating from their. She told them she knew I had been shot because I staggered back and recovered my balance. He said how fortunate not to have a big hole my chest. She then told me to tell how come the ball had only wrapped my ribs. Then told them drawing my bow back to shoot I had turned and had gotten my arrow off just as the ball wrapped me in the ribs. One of the woman said someone is looking out for you. Everyone chuckled at that comment. Jan said she'd wholeheartedly agreed. Then I spoke up and said it was Jan. She just gave me a poke on the arm shook her head rolling her eyes. This brought on another round of laughter. We said our goodbyes and rode through the village, was hard to believe how much it had expanded. Headed back to the farm for supper, the table was set and ready. Chuck and Chum were also there. They had been busy hauling lumber into the village. Chum mentioned he should make a trip to our trading post. It had been expanded a lot since first built. Told Chum I would make the trip if Jan was up to going Jan was more than willing.

A list had been sent back by the men running the post. One was Judd who had helped me recover our stolen goods. I decided to use a pack horse for our belongings and our comfort. My filly was still in excellent shape. Jan's horse had been hers for quite some time so we were comfortable with our mounts. We left crossing the river on a barge that had been built as a ferry. Chuck and Chum had invested in the project so our fair was free. We owned the biggest share of the barge. The two men who took care of it were more than happy with the results Chuck and Chum made sure they got their share and always a little more. This made for two good men

A Past Life: as told by Brave Hawk

handling the ferry. Large ropes were hooked to each end of the ferry. A team of horses on each side would pull the ferry back and forth. They had signals when everything was ready. Jan and I took our time to set up camp early at times, made love quite often. We just enjoyed our trip and each other.

When we arrived at the post Judd came out was glad to see us. He said had not had any problems since we had recovered our goods. Had quite a few Indian in for trading. I had informed them not to cheat the Indians. Jan I camped outside. We told Judd the goods were on their way. Judd said some were always looking for whiskey, they were getting used to being told we didn't trade in whiskey and had none. He had also let one chief in to show him there was none to be had. Most now didn't ask anymore. Was hoping to see some of my villagers come to the trading post. Judd said he had not seen them for quite a while. They had came in and made a big trade and he had not seen them since. We stayed for a week, the day before were to head back a chief and his entourage showed up for trade. He spotted me and said Brave Hawk very much smart kill off our trader now have to come in trade here with you. I didn't try to deny his words. Jan wanted to know what was being said. I wasn't about to lie to her. Told her he called me by name and told me I was smart to kill off his trader to force them to trade at our trading post. Had not told Jan or anyone in particular about what had happened. She then said did you really do that. I knew would have to tell her the whole story of how we had recovered our goods. How this man had been stealing from us then got greedy and had stolen our whole supply of goods. Judd and I had gotten them back. Yes I had killed this man but in self-defense. He was hunting me I was lucky and shot and didn't miss he did. And getting him first even though we had got a shot at me. Judd was listening and told her he had killed one of the men who was trying to kill me. Jan said I just knew you wouldn't just kill someone just for profit. I told her would have to tell her more about my Indian life. I let her know had killed only in self-defense.

Judd had talked to Jan when I was talking with the chief and some of their Braves. Asked if they had seen my brother or any of the trackers from my village. They hadn't seen any for some time. Then I found out the Bowman that had been sent to kill me was also there. They thought I would be very angry and try to kill him. He stood very proud and acknowledged it was he. I smiled and went to him and said I was very glad he had missed. This seemed to surprise him. I went and put my hands on his shoulders in a sign of friendship. He reciprocated with much relief. Even the chief was surprised at my ease and my comments. I found I had made another friend that would go out of his way for me. We then sat around a small fire and did a lot of talking. A lot of exaggeration also. They never did ask how I had knocked the arrows out of the air and I didn't tell them either. They all believed I was protected by a powerful spirit I apologize to Jan telling her when the men got together the woman at this time were not welcome. Was the Indian way. Jan had no problem with this she just wish he could understand what was being said. She said I can't believe how well you speak their language, told her that I had lived with them for some time as I had related before and that was all that was spoken so was forced to learn or be left out of everything..

Jan then said aren't you going to tell me about what happened. She said what went on between you and that one brave that looked very uncomfortable until you talk to him and put your hands on his shoulders, he then reciprocated. Then had to tell her he was their best Bowman and had been sent by his shaman but not his chief to kill me with his bow. My brother had yelled a warning I then knocked both arrows out of the air with my knife. Jan's next question how did you ever do that. Then had to tell her how I had found to do this from the time at the village not the Indian village. This is at our village, they were having a bow contest. I stood down by the targets to acknowledge the hits. Told the other two men I could knock an arrow out of the air and proceeded to do just that. The Man shooting the arrow was very upset. When he found out about my quote to the other men he was also amazed. If standing to

A Past Life: as told by Brave Hawk

the side you could see the arrow coming and if quick enough could knock it down. Jan said no wonder they respect you, not too many would be able to do that. I had not related any of the gory parts of my living with the Indians as yet. She heard them call me by name in Indian wanted to know what it meant in English. Jan could see I was uncomfortable in telling her. I was afraid I would have to tell her why. Finally decided to tell her, she was amazed at the name of Brave Hawk. She then said later you will have to tell me how they came to call you Brave Hawk. You always told everyone your name was Bird. I replied that's what everyone calls me. Jan laughed and said not these Indians, you had to do something to earn that name.

On our trip back to the farm, Jan's curiosity got the best of her. She finally said are you going to tell me how they come to call you Brave Hawk or will I have to pound on you. We both got to laughing. I then told her about the large Indian that came to the village and how everyone avoided him if possible. How he tried to get me to get him some food and I spit on him. My adopted mother and my Indian girlfriend stepped in to stop him from attacking me. But because of the insult would have to meet him in a battle to the death. Most didn't think I had a chance he had already killed six or eight in the same type of challenge. My adopted mother wanted me to leave also my girlfriend said she would leave with me. I had watched this brave and he was just an oversized bully. I would use Chuck's fighting instruction to best him. I told Jan I had a Tomahawk given me from the chief and my large knife I carried on my shoulder. When we met in the circle that had been drawn, I was the first to enter. He entered with a yell waving his Tomahawks, I made a few bounds and leaped into the air catching his Tomahawks with my left hand as I twisted drove my knife into his neck and down into his chest. I lit on my feet ready for him to turn and try to get me with his Tomahawks. He just dropped them and headed to the two Braves that he came with, dropping just outside the circle. The two Braves turned their backs on him and left. The other said was very brave to face him. When I attacked him it was like a hawk in for the kill. She then said it wasn't any worse than what you went through in the city. Also told her that shaman had assured my adopted mother and the chief I would come out victorious. She then asked what Chuck's instructions had been. Told her always make the first move and blow if possible his advice had probably saved my life.

Back to the farm, everything was running smoothly gardens and fields were producing well. The sawmill was going full blast. More orders that we could actually handle. We made the rounds and visits Chuck and Chum had claimed the lake and a lot of the land that was around we had surveyors lay out the land for a good mile around the lake with metal stakes at each corner. They had carpenters come up and redo and rebuild the cabin Jan and I were surprised to find how nice it was. Mom Chuck, Sue and Chum said it was their wedding gift to us we were both astounded. The deeds had been recorded in our names. Jan understood this much better than I did, never getting into the land rights and deeds. The complete farm consisted of around 1000 acres a lot of it was land. Our sawmill was on the border so most of the wood brought to the mill was on other land.

We finally decided to go to the city and see Jan's father and see how Guy and Bess were doing. Jan's father was glad to see us and he had to have a dinner for his friends and Guy and Bess's parents and friends. Jan said dad loves a good party and dinner. There had to be 20 or 30 people. We had sat down and had a glass of wine just before eating. Liquors if someone wanted such. A glass of wine was my limit, everybody was talking about the news of the day. What other business were doing etc. Someone asked has any one new news. Jan spoke up and said I have some, I wasn't expecting what she was about to relate to the guest. You all know my husband by the name he goes by Bird. She said the Bird the Indians call him is Brave Hawk. So now you know what kind of bird he is. She had a big grin on her face, all I could do was look at her and grin I shook my finger at her. This just made her laugh. I just hoped I wouldn't have to relate how the name was given. Guy and Bess were doing

A Past Life: As Told by Brave Hawk

real well. Guy's father had found someone to help out with running the business. He would take care of the financial part, the man he hired would take care of the shop. So Guy could go on the excursion to the West to meet my Indian family. Jan and I had made plans that were still in the process. We wanted it to be as comfortable as possible. We would need just the bare essentials a few pots and pans for cooking each carrying Flint for starting fires. Jan asked why each carry Flint. I answered just an insurance if anyone lost their flint one of us would have one. Fire was one of our basic needs and kept the bugs off in the evening and at night did our cooking and would keep us warm if need be. Frying pans and a pot for making stew we would be living mostly off the land and would have to scrounge for food. I knew of a lot of the edible plants because of all my excursions with native woman they had told me about a lot of the plants and what they were good for and which were edible.

Jan and I spent a lot of time at the lake. Decided to make up some wooden pipe to pipe the water into the cabin. Had already located a spring, would damn up and bury the wooden pipe in the ground. At the sawmill had wood lathe to turn pillars in post with different designs. Used this to make the pipe. We saw them in two then gouge out the center, then put them back together was strapped with metal bands. The ends had been turned to fit together snugly. Wasn't very long we had spring water in the cabin. We had done this at the farm years before. It had been improved on by Chuck and Chum. We had the only home around with running water in the house. Our faucets were made of wood with metal handles.

The village and expanded quite a lot everyone seemed be doing quite well. The Sunday games were still going on, Jan I would go and just observe. Jan and I had thought about getting into the running contest. Looked like a lot of competition, some of the villagers remembered me as their best runner and had beaten all other competitors. They prodded me into giving it a try, I was still in good running shape. Hadn't quit running even though I rode a horse a lot. I knew Jan also like to run. The village had expanded being twice the size or larger. A lot of strangers and some looked like they could really run. There apparel suggested they were ready for running. The village had set up short runs and one very long run. The long run gave the best prize, so most were holding out for the long run myself included. Jan entered the shorter runs and won two out of the four runs. Placing second in the other two. The run I was waiting for was 2 miles or a little more, some over a rugged terrain. We started out most with a big rush. Just stayed back to keep track of who was going to be out front. Found I was running at an easy pace for me, stayed back until the front runners picked up their pace and started to leave the slower behind, I just pass them with not much effort. When we got to the halfway mark there were only nine or 10 up front this is when I decided to move up to the front two runners. Still wasn't crowding myself as yet. When with the Indians had run all day and not stop till late in the afternoon or evening. So this didn't seem a big challenge for me. The front two runners glanced back and found me at their heels, they again picked up the pace. One started to lag back I passed him, found I would be competing with just one man. Stayed with him all the way, we were way ahead of all the other runners. The last quarter-mile he started to really push. Let him stay a step ahead, then really push myself to pass him for the finish. When crossing the finish line I was 50 or more paces in front of him. I pulled up and caught my breath but wasn't overly tired. He came across a line and took him quite a while to get his wind back. He then came over to me and congratulated me telling me he had never been beaten before.

Told him about running with the Indians. How most could out run me, they could run all day I was able to do the same but would be tired out. They seem not to tire anywhere near as much. I didn't have much use for the prize and offered it to him. He was reluctant to take it but I insisted so he finally accepted. Jan came over and also congratulated me then introduced him to Jan. He said he had watched her run and said if she had been able to rest between races he believe she would have won all she had entered.

A Past Life: as told by Brave Hawk

Mom and Sue were surprised to see Jan run in the contest. Very few woman ever entered the running contest. She had out run all the men and two other girls had ran, also did quite well. Mom and Sue congratulated both of us at our wins. They knew a lot more of the villagers than we did. Had been away just long enough to have the village expand to better than twice its size. Mom and Sue introduced us to quite a few of the people. There were some that were good friends others were customers. This was really good for our business. Everyone enjoyed the games and the contest. Found Chuck, Mom, Chum and Sue donated a lot of the prizes and food.

Chuck and Chum were in the city taking care of a lot of the business. Buying things for trade and sale at the village also to trade with the Indians. Found that beads were highly prized by the Indians also pots pans, Tomahawk's now they wanted rifles. We had not traded rifles as yet. Once Chuck and Chum found a supplier with reasonable prices on them we would more than likely start using them in our trading. The Arapahoe were so good with a bow didn't see them going to the rifle. I use my bow more than I did the rifle. Took a lot of time and practice to be an excellent shot. I now could bring down a grouse in flight.

We all headed back to the farm. Mom and Sue had given the day off to all the help, we would have to make a quick meal of whatever we could find. We were all surprised to have a meal cooked and waiting for us. Our cook and maids had planned ahead and came back earlier to get the meal ready. Mom and Sue thank them and said it was their day off, they didn't have to do this. Their answer was they had to eat to.

Fall season came a lot of getting ready for winter. Harvesting crops and storing. Our barns were full we always seem to have a good harvest. Our people working for us were very reliable. The horses and cows were well cared for, it was hard for me to picture the original farm and how much we had expanded. Winter months card games and checkers a lot of different games were played especially on Sundays very little turmoil. Enjoyed the winter outdoors did a lot of walking looking for the different animal tracks, also the sledding when enough snow. The helps children were a pleasure to have around. Growing up there were no children around for me. Chum was my only companion. Didn't get to play with children until I was with my Indian family. The Braves didn't play like kids the way I did. This endeared me that much more to them especially the woman.

Jan and I would make trips to the cabin at the lake just for the peace and quiet and to enjoy each other. Jan and Bess were somehow practicing birth control. They didn't want to be pregnant on our Western excursion. Mom and Sue had recommend some type of herb Jan had heard about it from some sources in the city. Most men had no idea of this.

We were spending a lot of time at the cabin fall weather was very pleasant. The boat was a nice addition and made fishing much easier and let us a get away from the shore. Not near as many bugs out on the lake. Told Jan would like to catch a really big trout, she thought we already had. Our hooks were handmade took a lot of patience to make them. Early afternoon Jan asked when we were going out on the lake. We would go after dark this is when the large fish usually feed. Shortly after supper and nightfall put the boat into the lake. Told Jan to listen we would hear the big ones near the surface feeding on the bugs sometimes sounded like they were sucking them in. Decided To let Jan have a try. She cast the line out with a hook and lure, no more than hit the water and a big one hit almost pulling the poll out of Jan's hands. She stood up quick and almost upended the boat. The fish was very large finally got it up near the boat and I grabbed it in the gills and into the boat. Jan's, said wow. Then she said she had been doubtful of my telling her the big fish fed at night. How did I ever find this out. Related my Indian friends had taught me this also how to catch them by hand if need be. This also took a lot of time and patience. We did this mostly in the streams. Much harder to do in the lake. We use spears

A Past Life: as told by Brave Hawk

also had some made with a kind of hooked branch this was used after spearing to pull them into the canoe hunting and fishing was their way of life at this time so I learned a lot from them. Especially from my tracker friend Gonacheaw.

Next morning Jan wanted to head back to the farm with this big trout. She said we've just got to show it to everyone. Chum and I had caught a lot of fish but like the smaller ones for eating. The lake was only 5 to 8 acres so could be fished out with a lot of fishing pressure. We had cut a swath around the lake and warned it to be private land. We had caught some in with nets catching fish, this is when we put a stop to anyone fishing. Indicated the trail in with signs anyone caught would be prosecuted. Headed back to the farm, we had gotten up early so everyone was just finishing breakfast. The roosters were still crowing when we came in. Jan lugging the big trout. Everyone was amazed at the size of it. The spots were as big as some of the coins we used for trading. Chuck and Chum Were Back from the City and both chuckled at Jan's excitement. Chum's comment was like mine the smaller ones were better eating. Jan got a lot of compliments on her catch. A lot of the city woman, younger girls her age would be very envious of her. Young girls at the farm asked weren't we afraid to go out fishing in the dark. Jan said using, my Indian name, Brave Hawk was with me nothing to be afraid of. This got a big chuckle out of Chuck and Chum. We then had our breakfast. Mom and Sue were getting everyone to their assigned chores. Our hen-house had been tripled in size so gathering eggs was another chore the girls enjoyed.

Talking to Chuck and Chum I had mentioned the cabin was great. I then said was going to make a larger boat. They just laughed and said they had plans but hadn't got to it yet.

When at the cabin had seen sign of bear, they had been around the cabin. They hadn't broken in as yet. I decided to hunt them again before they did break in. Jan was excited and wasn't about to be left out. She thought we would track them. I told her that was too time-consuming. We would put out bait and entice them in. I would be a lot more cautious and make sure not be caught off guard again. Took a few days after putting out the bait before they started to come to it. Had set up our lean to on the downwind side on a rise so we would be looking down at the site. When we had the bears coming we then sat in our lean to. This time had viewing on both sides and back. Being caught off guard once was more than enough. Jan and Bess were both very good rifle shot's. Jan's father had insisted on her and Bess to learn to handle a rifle. Not just to shoot but reload and shoot again if need be. Both girls had been tomboy's so are used to a little rough-and-tumble. By the signs we are seeing more than one bear was coming to the bait. The days were very pleasant. Sitting in the lean to wasn't very uncomfortable. Started to get dark and Jan thought we would leave. I just shook my head no. Motioned to her a while yet. No more than settled back down when we see movement. Two bears ambled into the feed could see Jan was very excited. She had the rifle and I had my bow. Had told her to shoot first then I would follow with a shot from my bow. Jan's bear made a big jump and had started to run. I knew it was hit hard. The bear I shot with my bow was chewing on the arrow feathers. Had another arrow knocked just in case would need another shot. Also had Jan reload her rifle. I was sure Jan's bear wasn't going very far either. Waiting for Jan to reload and prime her rifle. Let things calm down, and went over to the arrowed bear he was dead. Could see the other bears trail and begin to follow it, didn't go very far when a bear raised up in front of us I put my arrow into his chest, Jan was just behind me and heard and also saw the bear raise up. She stepped to my side and also fired into the bear as he was chewing on the arrow. This put him down for good. I was surprised and was sure that the bear Jan had shot was hit real hard. Looking at the tracks found Jan's bear just a short distance in front of us this was the third bear. We ended up with three good-sized bears. I told Jan I would gut the bears out but we would need help getting them back. She went got her horse and went for help. Wasn't long but was getting quite dark by this time. I had gotten my pony and had drug all three bears to the cabin which wasn't too

A Past Life: as told by Brave Hawk

far from the lean to. Could hear them coming they had brought a to wheel cart. Much easier to maneuver on the trail. We were able to get all three bear in to the cart. My pony was used to the hunting and odors. The other ponies were quite antsy from the smell. Got them calm down and were on our way. This was a lot better than the hog that had been butchered earlier. We all liked bear meat.

All the bears were very fat, so rendered fat into useful things for cooking and for candles etc. We all had a good meal next evening. A lot of it was smoked in our smokehouse in and cured with salt. Some was pickled in our pickling barrels. We wouldn't have to butcher one of the young bulls we were raising for this purpose. All had to hear about our adventure. Jan telling the tale made it a lot more exciting than I could have. Especially when the third bear had risen up in front of us. I then decided to let her tell about any of our other escapades.

Found a lot of the men wouldn't venture into the woods at night. Jan was amazed at me for not being afraid of the woods at night. She and I had ventured out quite often just to hear and see the night goings on. A lot of the animals forged at night. One thing I found we both had good night vision. Most of the man and woman had to have a lantern even on a good trail. We both could see better without the lantern. They couldn't get over Jan out hunting with me. Some of the older woman didn't think it right. Mom was a little upset at first but Sue took it right in stride. Telling everyone that Jan was one of the new woman coming of age. This seemed to calm them down. A couple of the older ladies had a way of shunning Jan. The younger girls would engaged Jan whenever they could, Asking all kinds of questions, who had taught her to shoot a rifle, did she like to hunt. Jan knew a lot of the girls would never get the opportunity to shoot or hunt. She would talk to them and also tell them she also loved to cook and sew. Jan and Aunt Sue became very close. Jan said Sue could calm any situation she just had the calmness personality and intelligence to tackle any situation and resolve it.

Our farm had become almost a small village. Mill hands and wife had houses also the farm help. The maids" stayed in our large house had rooms of their own. How it had expanded since I was a child. Mom and Sue took care of the books and finances. Chuck and Chum were the overseers of the whole enterprise. Our garden was a communal affair everyone mostly the woman were working and keeping the weeds out and also the varmints away .We now had a couple of dogs that did a good job of that.

Fall progressed into winter, a lot less work for most. Chickens had to be fed, cows horses were out most of the time to forge. We also supplemented their feed. The winter went by with a lot of card playing and games of different sort. A lot of sewing for spring clothes, cotton linens and fine wool made for the best garments. Wool at the time was the least expensive. We now could afford all three and had amassed a large quantity. The old mule had died during the winter just from old age. We had excellent help so everything went smoothly. The sawmill ran most of the winter. The stream froze over and would shut things down for a while. Would warm up and things would go again. Jan and I were making plans for our excursion to see my Indian family with Bess and Guy. aunt Sue was really interested she helped with our plans, myself I would have no problem going alone.

Sue mentioned it would be nice to accompany you on this trip. Jan and I both were surprise, both chimed in at the same time why don't you come with us. She said the furthest she had been was to the city. Had never been on an exciting excursion like we were planning. We then asked her about Chum what he thought about her idea and would he also want to come along. He had said he had gone as far west as he wanted, the trading post was keeping him busy also overseeing the sawmill. He was all for Sue going. He said with Bird running the trip he wouldn't have much to worry about. This really excited Jan and myself. Sue would make a wonderful addition to our excursion. She said I just need something like this to be able to tell everyone about this excursion. Her woman friends she knew would be envious, but would be thrilled to have her relate what everything was like. She especially wanted to meet my Indian family.

Mom at first wasn't too enthused. Knowing mom she would encourage rather than discourage Sue. Chum told me you take good care of my Sue. I know you will Bird without me having to tell you to.

We again decided to go into the city for a visit with Jan's dad and Bess' and Guy's parents. Jan's dad had a dinner laid out for a couple of evenings later. This would be a get together for the families. After a good dinner we were all sitting and discussing our excursion. Jan's dad said he would be the first to go but he was just too old now. Guy and Bess' dad said the same thing. Bess' mom wasn't at all happy about her going. Guy said this is to be our honeymoon trip. Bess' mom said, the Indians will probably do all of you in. I then told her my Indian family were not hostile to us and would go out of their way to protect us. I also knew the Indians would be fascinated with Jan's hair it was almost blond, Bess was a redhead so that would be as fascinating for the Indians also. I didn't dare tell this at the dinner talk. Bess' mom would have been very upset. When Guy and Bess heard Sue was also coming they were amazed at first. Sue really wasn't that much older than what we were. She was a welcome companion.

Everything was set for the spring, I told the woman bring just the bare essentials. Taken a lot of extras would be a burden in the long run. Bess came back to the farm with us. The three girls were making their plans and just what to take and what they would need. I felt we would be gone for 2 to 3 months more or less. Soap was one of their priorities. Towels and clothes etc. We would take traveling food but would not use it only if we had to. Food in the spring was plentiful if you knew what to look for. One tent big enough to sleep all five especially in bad weather. If we pack something and found we didn't need it we would leave it behind. They laughed at this,

Aunt Sue grinned and nodded. She knew other girls were taking too much cosmetics etc.

Aunt Sue designed some woman's outer pants. She had worn them around the farm. Some were made of the finest wool others were made of cotton and some of the linen. She told the girls the bugs couldn't get up and bite you on the rear. This got a big laugh out of the girls and mom. Mom said leave it to Sue to think of doing it the best way.

Bess road side-saddle, most of the city woman of the upper crust rode this way. Jan and Sue both wouldn't ride side saddle, told darn uncomfortable for a long ride. Jan and Sue were on the same way of thinking. Comfort and protection both. So mom Sue Jan Bess made up outfits just for our excursions West. Some of the villagers thought it disgrace to where mens pants. Aunt Sue had the answer, these are not mens pants they are woman's, she also stated what was a different between the split skirt except for more floppy material. Sue Jan and Bess wore them even in the village. The younger girls started to do the same. Startled a lot of the men and some though it just awful. Most men accepted the idea. A lot of their woman had wore pants but never wore them in the village.

Made a few trips back into the city to get trading supplies to help. Chuck and Chum. The girls and Aunt Sue made the dinners. Everyone wanted to hear about our Western excursion. Jan and Bess were really excited and showed their enthusiasm in the telling of how they were getting ready. Bess also stated she was no longer riding side-saddle. All their friends were envious. But were glad for the girls and Sue. I was really appreciated of, the influence Sue was having on the girls. She was making them cut back to the bare essentials. I talked to Chuck and Chum, they both agreed. I had enough experience to keep us out of trouble. My Indian family would accept me with no problems. There were always renegades both Indian and white men, mostly white men. Just prayed would not run into either on our trip. Back at the farm. Mom was also getting things together. Also some goods for trading. A lot of beads etc. We planned on nine or 10 horses and all the ones we road and the others were packing gear and gifts for the Indian family. We were almost ready to go.

Printed in the USA
CPSIA information can be obtained
at www.ICGtesting.com
LVHW020800130124
768547LV00102B/186